One Nation under AARP

One Nation under AARP

The Fight over Medicare, Social Security, and America's Future

Frederick R. Lynch

UNIVERSITY OF CALIFORNIA PRESS

Berkeley   Los Angeles   London

University of California Press, one of the most distinguished university presses in the United States, enriches lives around the world by advancing scholarship in the humanities, social sciences, and natural sciences. Its activities are supported by the UC Press Foundation and by philanthropic contributions from individuals and institutions. For more information, visit www.ucpress.edu.

University of California Press
Berkeley and Los Angeles, California

University of California Press, Ltd.
London, England

Library of Congress Cataloging-in-Publication Data

Lynch, Frederick R.
    One nation under AARP : the fight over medicare, social security, and America's future / Frederick R. Lynch.
        p.   cm.
    Includes bibliographical references and index.
    ISBN 978-0-520-25653-8 (cloth : alk. paper)
    ISBN 978-0-520-26828-9 (pbk. : alk. paper)
    1. Senior power—United States.   2. Older people—Political activity—United States.   3. Baby boom generation—United States.   4. American Association of Retired Persons .   I. Title.
    HQ1064.U5L94 2011
    306.3'80973—dc22   2010037306

Manufactured in the United States of America

19 18 17 16 15 14 13 12 11
10 9 8 7 6 5 4 3 2 1

This book is printed on Cascades Enviro 100, a 100% post consumer waste, recycled, de-inked fiber. FSC recycled certified and processed chlorine free. It is acid free, Ecologo certified, and manufactured by BioGas energy.

Once again:
For my sister, Peg
And the memory of our parents

CONTENTS

ACKNOWLEDGMENTS

Many thanks to stalwart friends and colleagues Gary Jason, Jack Pitney, Jan Allard, Monica Morris, David Sadava, Bill Frey, Ralph Rossum, Joe Cardoza, Jonathan Tilove, and a very special colleague and pal, the late Judith Merkle. I very much appreciate Greg O'Neill, H.R. "Rick" Moody, Bob Binstock, and Rob Hudson welcoming me into the ranks of gerontologists. John Rother and many others at AARP were extremely generous with time and insights.

My editor at UC Press, Naomi Schneider, was wonderfully supportive in reading numerous chapter drafts and, above all, extremely patient in providing generous deadline extensions to incorporate the unpredictable, unfolding developments of 2008 and 2010 that have proved so crucial in the saga of aging boomers, AARP, and the coming entitlement battles. Elisabeth Magnus was a tireless, sharp-eyed copy editor. My literary agent, Jill Marsal, facilitated my getting together with UC Press. I've also been aided by able student assistants, Matt Horwitz, Alison Strother, and Reed MacPhail.

I am grateful for several grants sustaining the research over the years. More than a decade ago, the Sarah Scaife Foundation provided valuable seed money for this research, as did the Earhart Foundation. More recently, I was aided by several smaller grants from Claremont

McKenna College research institutes, including the Benjamin Z. Gould Center, the Berger Institute for the Study of Work, Family, and Children, and the Office of the Dean of Faculty.

Former Claremont McKenna College president Jack Stark, current president Pamela B. Gann, deans Anthony Fucaloro, Jerry Garris, and Gregory Hess, and Government Department chair Ralph Rossum provided academic sanctuary for a politically incorrect sociologist. And a special salute to Jonathan Knight, former director of the American Association of University Professors' Office of Academic Freedom, Tenure and Governance—whose legal acumen and blunt e-mails helped ensure that "sanctuary" finally became "tenure."

.　　.　　.

Portions of chapters 2 through 4 appeared in abbreviated form in "Political Power and the Baby Boomers" in editor Robert Hudson's The New Politics of Old Age Policy, 2nd ed., © The Johns Hopkins University Press. Expanded and updated reprinting with permission of The Johns Hopkins University Press.

Quotation of the television interview of Bill Clinton by Charlie Rose is by permission of The Charlie Rose Show.

Quotation of David Walker and a listener on the Diane Rehm Show is by permission of National Public Radio's The Diane Rehm Show from WAMU-FM in Washington, D.C.

Introduction

Not Going Quietly

It wasn't like, "Here's the political thing, here's the cultural thing." It was all woven together in the same sort of rebellious rock and roll attitude. When you said rock and roll, you didn't mean just the music. You meant it as a way of life, as a coat of armor against everything that was coming at you. It was a force to be reckoned with.

—Michael Moore (2007)

We honored our part of the bargain. We are counting on the amounts reported to us on our Social Security forms. If this contract is broken, there will be hell to pay from a generation that knows how to organize and inflict political pain.

—Letter to the editor, *Washington Post* (August 20, 2002)

On an October Friday night in 2006, the rock band "Splash!"—whose members were in their twenties and thirties—loudly belted out hits of the 1960s and 1970s. Most of the four hundred or so people listening and dancing to the music were in their fifties and early sixties—aging baby boomers who did not necessarily think of themselves or their music as "golden oldies." Yet this musical happening at California's Anaheim Convention Center was hosted by AARP, part of a three-day "Life @ 50+" megaconference that drew twenty-five thousand registered attendees.

The Anaheim megaconference would be one of the smoothest, most successful—and certainly the most star-studded—of these annual events, which had begun with a mere six thousand attendees at the first Life @ 50+ gathering in Dallas in 2001. And, befitting the Disneyland slogan of the "happiest place on earth," the 2006 event may have been the most upbeat and carefree of all such gatherings before and since. Under the blue skies and golden California sun, the 2000–2002 "Dot-Com Crash" had become a dim memory, while the gathering thunderclouds of the coming real estate meltdown, stock market crash, and "Great Recession" were still not yet on the horizon.

A primary purpose of these entertainment-and-merchandizing extravaganzas is to demonstrate to fifty-plus boomers that the nation's largest senior citizen lobby is no longer their parents' AARP. A "rebranded" forty-million-member AARP is actively recruiting seventy-eight million graying baby boomers (born 1946–64). The mating dance of these organizational and generational giants has enormous implications for the nation's political future. Just under half the voters in the 2008 and 2010 elections were over age fifty; approximately half of those voters were also members of AARP, the nation's fourth-highest-spending lobbying organization from 1998 to 2009. Not since the heyday of America's industrial unions has there been such a potential concentration of member-based organizational clout. And this development remains completely unstudied.

The relatively few books about boomers chronicle their contentious past. This one is about their even more problematic economic, political, and sociological future. Boomers will not go gently into that good night. As young adults, an educated boomer vanguard wrought considerable political and social change. Forty years later, boomers are again politically restive. Historic real estate and stock market declines have made large numbers of them economically vulnerable just as they approach voluntary (or forced) retirement and old age. As a group, aging boomers are not financially prepared for retirement and old age; they are going to be more dependent upon Medicare and Social Security than they'd ever assumed. They are also politically and culturally vulnerable; they are not well liked; as a generation they are often self-critical and apologetic: stereotypes abound.

Long postponed, an epic political fight over changes in Medicare and Social Security is being forced by the ballooning national debt. If aging boomers are to protect these entitlements, they will need leaders, friends, and allies. The most likely all-in-one candidate is AARP.

One Nation under AARP examines three key issues. First, there is the question of boomers' "senior power" potential. Are aging boomers a sleeping political giant? The steep stock market and real estate declines, followed by the Great Recession, raised boomers' age awareness and retirement anxieties. Threatened cutbacks in pensions, Social Security, and Medicare could produce a higher degree of age and generational consciousness, activating latent senior power in the form of a boomer voting bloc or more organized political movements. The onset of any such mobilization, I think, is more likely among Older Boomers (born during 1946–55) than Younger Boomers (born during 1956–64), because the former are closest to retirement and most economically vulnerable. Older Boomers, therefore, are the primary focus of this book.

Highly educated Older Boomers have an activist heritage: they were the backbone of the 1960s protest movements. If fading Golden Years visions are further threatened by cutbacks in Medicare, Social Security, and also public and private pensions, it is reasonable to assume that the generation that "knows how to organize and inflict political pain" might revive its activist heritage with the modern organizational tools of the Web and the Internet—but only if aging boomers can overcome their trademark "do your own thing" culture of individualism, competitiveness, and mistrust of government, as well as their deep demographic and political divides.

The relationship between seventy-eight million aging boomers and the forty-million-member AARP is a second major focus of this book. AARP (which shed its older title of American Association of Retired Persons because more than half of its members are *not* retired) must necessarily stimulate boomers' age awareness to entice them into becoming members and purchasing AARP's products and services. Though they generally take care to avoid labeling "boomers" as such, AARP nonetheless is flooding boomers' mailboxes—and raising their consciousness—about both the vulnerabilities and positive potential of senior citizenship.

Yet AARP's leaders are reluctant to champion a boomer-centric politics that might prove polarizing or unpredictable or, worse, might reinforce critics' AARP stereotype as the "greedy geezers'" political lobby. Instead, under the leadership of the former CEO Bill Novelli and the current leader A. Barry Rand, a more inclusively inclined AARP is more likely to broker aging boomers' interests, balancing them with those of other groups as the giant organization expands its mission of broader societal change for "everyone who has a birthday." AARP is increasingly studying the needs and desires of the next generation of senior citizens—now in their thirties and forties. More cynical AARP watchers suspect that the organization's drive to maximize membership, sell insurance, and provide other services trumps its willingness to take bold political stands. Liberals have long been frustrated by AARP's refusal to lobby for a single-payer, Canadian-style health care system; conversely, conservatives have always suspected AARP's leaders are liberals bent on furthering "socialized medicine."

Thus the third issue examined extensively throughout *One Nation under AARP* is how aging boomers and AARP are negotiating an increasingly competitive, globalized "supercapitalism," major demographic changes, and the rise of a "Post-American World." Both boomers and AARP were created in the mid-twentieth-century era of the nation-state and a strong sense of national unity, trust, and civic ties forged by World War II and sustained by a thirty-year cold war. But the growth of global supercapitalism with its unpredictable economic crises, mass migrations, and the rise of new economic powers such as China and India herald greater international influence, integration, and regulation.[1]

The 2008 presidential elections revealed that responses to globalization and other issues are strongly structured by a deep societal divide marked by class, education, and culture. On the one hand, millions of older middle- and working-class Americans feel economically threatened by globalization—especially those without college degrees who reside in regions affected by overseas outsourcing and/or high immigration levels. Indeed, blue-collar workers (especially men) have been hardest hit in the current recession. They tend to be patriotic nationalists and look to the nation-state for both economic and military protection.

On the other hand, the nation's political, economic, and cultural elites, as well as many members of its highly educated professional and managerial classes, embrace the new international "post-American" order. Many of the nation's top leaders are also considered members of a "New Global Elite"—as portrayed in a special double issue of *Newsweek* in late 2008.[2] First and foremost on the *Newsweek* global elite roster was President Barack Obama, who has many times referred to himself as a "citizen of the world." This label resonates well with an Obama core campaign constituency of younger, more ethnically diverse Americans. Indeed, the pollster John Zogby characterizes younger Americans as the "First Global Generation" who "defer less to American values . . . and see themselves as citizens of the planet, not of any nation in particular."[3]

The advent of a new global order poses a fundamental dilemma for national entitlements that the nation's elites and the general public have refused to recognize: Social Security, Medicare, and other old-age entitlements are based on the sociological and cultural foundation of the nation-state. But national borders, the emotionally based sense of identity, loyalty, national community, the intergenerational compact, and the spirit of *E Pluribus Unum* risk erosion through supercapitalism, rising inequality, mass immigration, multiculturalism, increased international work and travel, the Internet and World Wide Web, and decreasing involvement with local groups, civic associations, and communities.[4]

The absence of leadership and a "functioning national group" to discuss such matters troubles National Public Radio commentator Dick Meyer and many others. He complains that in a fragmented, balkanized America, "What is missing is a leadership or inspiration *across* groups. By definition, there cannot be a leader without a functioning group of followers. There is no functioning national group in America today."[5]

AARP wants to answer this call, to both lead and build a national forum to address issues of generational equity in a changing world. To do so, AARP has been changing itself and broadening its mission. For the past decade, it has conducted an organizational makeover. The initial, primary goal of this "brand enhancement" has been to attract and retain large numbers of reluctantly aging baby boomers.

ROMANCING THE BOOMERS

The organizers of AARP's annual "Life @ 50+" conferences realize that the best route to boomers' wallets, hearts, and minds is through the music and popular culture of their youth. At the 2006 Anaheim Life @ 50+ megaconference, "Splash!" provided classic rock and pop at the largest of AARP's "Studio 50+ Nightclubs." Two other smaller ballrooms featured songs from Motown's 1960s heyday and another blared "Latin fusion." Earlier in the day the convention amphitheater was packed to watch a well-preserved Raquel Welch (age sixty-five) discuss secrets for remaining youthful. At other times, Dan Rather and Connie Chung talked about news and current events. Maya Angelou read poetry. The actress Ruby Dee discussed civil rights. The comedienne Joan Rivers interviewed conference goers. Bill Cosby and Jose Feliciano provided Friday evening entertainment. And Saturday night was more than all right for Elton John, who performed for a sold-out crowd of ten thousand people.

Yet beneath the three-day festival of nostalgia, music, dancing, and upbeat lectures were grim reminders of a new era of generational angst: the forever young generation cannot stop the clock.

Boomers are becoming increasingly vulnerable to health and financial setbacks.

A competitive, optimistic, fiercely individualistic generation is pondering aging and mortality. "Big Chill" moments multiply. "This is the cruelty of middle age," observed *New York Times* columnist Judith Warner. "I find: just when things have gotten good—really, really, consistently good—I have become aware that they will end."[6]

Two of the "Fab Four" Beatles are long deceased—as are several other famous singers from the rock-and-roll era. Those who survive and continue to perform are looking their age. Advertisements for medical services and pharmaceuticals proliferate. Boomers are experimenting with new funeral formats.

The powerful and wealthy are not immune. Bill Clinton, typified as the "first boomer" president, has had heart bypass surgery and wears a hearing aid. The second boomer president, George W. Bush, famously compulsive about fitness and exercise, nonetheless discovered he must undergo colonoscopies every three years because of the discovery of suspicious polyps. Tony Snow, Bush's youthful-looking press secretary, very publicly fought and ultimately lost a battle with colon cancer at age fifty-three. Snow died just weeks before Tim Russert, the popular television host of NBC's *Meet the Press,* dropped dead of a heart attack at age fifty-eight. And the pace and number of famous boomer mortalities would quicken daily, indeed, hourly.

Rank-and-file boomers were also encountering more medical tests, paying higher copayments for more prescription drugs, and coping with swiftly rising health insurance premiums. Even before the 2008 precipitous declines in the stock market and residential real estate, many boomers had saved very little for their retirement years. Millions of boomer "sandwich" families felt squeezed by trying simultaneously to save for retirement, to pay their kids' college tuition, and perhaps also to care for aging parents. The latter activity offers some troubling premonitions. While lovingly caring for her elderly mother, a single, childless boomer paused to ponder the likely loneliness of her own latter years in a much-read AARP *My Generation* magazine article: "Who Will Be 'Me' for Me?"[7]

AARP knows all this. Through dozens of surveys and hundreds of focus groups, no other organization has so thoroughly researched and studied the boomers. No other institution is as attuned to their preferences and future needs. Indeed, AARP anchors a proliferating services complex of medical, nonprofit, commercial, and government agencies geared to aging Americans. They have a rich and growing target. A 2006 Focalyst survey of thirty thousand Americans over the age of forty-two (half of all Americans) found that they control more than 90 percent of the nation's wealth, spend $3 trillion annually, and cast more than half of the votes in the 2004 national elections. (Indeed, according to CNN exit polls, voters over age forty constituted 64 percent of the 2008 national electorate.)[8]

The expanding supermarket of products and services for aging Americans was on display in the four hundred exhibits filling the Anaheim Convention Center's cavernous Exhibition Hall. The sprawling AARP Pavilion dominated the entrance. Its booths featured AARP insurance partnerships: AARP Medicare Supplemental Insurance and AARP Pharmacy Services (both administered by United Health Care), AARP Auto/Home Insurance (Hartford Insurance), AARP Life Insurance (New York Life), AARP Long-Term Care Insurance (MetLife), and AARP Mobile Home Insurance (Foremost). AARP Financial Services offered a Visa card (through First USA Bank) and new mutual funds designed for low- and middle-income investors (managed by State Street Bank). Other booths showcased AARP's nonprofit activities: AARP Community Service Leadership, AARP Foundation, the AARP Advocacy Bus (which toured the nation promoting AARP's issues), AARP Grassroots and Elections, the Voices of Civil Rights Project, and AARP's National Retired Teachers Association. Corporate America was there. Anheuser Busch, Home Depot, United Health Group, and Walgreens were the event's "platinum sponsors." Professional associations provided information about hospice and about chronic conditions such as alcoholism, Alzheimer's disease, heart disease, and macular degeneration. The American Cancer Society offered an especially graphic experience: a large, walk-through plastic replica of a human colon (with tumors).

Conventioneers mingled around the booths sponsored by the two largest government entitlement programs, the Centers for Medicare and Medicaid and the Social Security Administration. But the information provided there gave no indication that these popular, taken-for-granted programs constitute the financial and political time bombs of the twenty-first century. Seventy-eight million aging baby boomers will severely test the fiscal futures of Social Security and, especially, Medicare.

BOOMERS' SENIOR POWER POTENTIAL

Boomers' sheer numbers have been their source of power, impact, and identity. As they age, their generational clout may be magnified further by accrued wealth and political power. In 1999, *Age Power* author Ken Dychtwald predicted that boomers would continue the nation's trend toward economic and political gerontocracy. But how cohesive and well organized is this gerontocracy?[9]

Time magazine cover story reporter Daniel Okrent more darkly prophesied that "the size of the boomer generation and the tendency of the elderly to vote in greater percentages than any other age will converge to create a daunting political force . . . a gerontocracy of such unity and might that it will either utterly dominate the American political map or promote all-out generational warfare."[10] Former U.S. commerce secretary Peter Peterson, currently chairman of the powerful Blackstone investment firm and author of *Gray Dawn* and other demographic doomsday scenarios, has long prophesied that boomers' demands on Social Security and Medicare will mortgage the fiscal futures of their children. (His message is now amplified by the new Peter G. Peterson Foundation.)[11]

Aging boomers' senior power potential will depend upon whether age and generational identity transcend other social divisions. As with many other large groups, cohesive political action may fragment along the lines of class, ethnicity, gender, region, and religion. As mentioned in the previous section, class and education divide boomers and other Americans in their responses to globalization, multiculturalism, and changing demographics. This "wine-track/beer track" fault line among boomers—along with potent negative stereotypes of each group—widened during the 2008 presidential election and was especially visible in the Democratic primaries.

Boomers' senior power potential also depends upon two basic social psychological processes that facilitate mobilization and social movement formation. First, preexisting or socially constructed *consensus* among potential movement members on basic values, attitudes, and norms facilitates communication, interaction, and cohesion. Boomers' values and ideology emphasize individualism, competitiveness, and mistrust of major institutions (including government); this clearly inhibits large-scale collective mobilization. There is greater potential for mobilization with regard to a second variable fostering collective behavior: *convergence* upon similar economic interests, especially when reinforced by shared background characteristics—such as similarities in age, race, gender, and religion.[12]

Nothing unites a group like an external threat—especially one magnified by a major crisis. Thus the deep 2007–10 so-called Great Recession has forced recognition among boomers that a majority of them are financially "at risk" for their old age—at least 40 percent of them were financially ill prepared for retirement *before* the real estate and market meltdowns of 2008.[13]

Into this atmosphere of crisis and doubt, the new Obama White House and heavily Democratic Congress injected another political controversy: major health care/ Medicare reform. Voters over age fifty were the most opposed to this narrowly successful legislation. Controversial health care reform, rising public and private levels of debt, and bailouts of corporations by the government were, evidently, "precipitating events" for significant numbers of anxious or threatened Older Boomers via the still fluid "Tea Party" movement. Indeed, economic strain and turmoil combined with record-low levels of trust are classic sociological conditions that give rise to political or social protest movements.[14] A more direct catalyst or precipitating event for activating boomers' senior power—and a possible alliance with AARP—would be serious White House or congressional proposals to change Social Security or Medicare.

In *Boom!*, his 1960s retrospective, the veteran NBC anchor Tom Brokaw suggested that boomers should be willing to delay or forego some entitlement benefits.[15] More recently, Michael Kinsley proposed in an *Atlantic* magazine cover story that aging boomers should subject themselves to a new, low-threshold inheritance tax to reduce the national debt burden for younger generations.[16] But George Anders, a Pulitzer Prize–winning health care reporter for the *Wall Street Journal*, suggested a more likely response to entitlement cutbacks or demands for generational atonement. "Boomers," he told me, "have a habit of saying 'no' to 'no.'"[17]

The arguments for and against "boomer power" (age-based consciousness with potential for expression as a voting bloc or political movement) are a dialectical, ongoing theme throughout this book.

Social Insecurity and the Risk-Shift Dilemma

For nearly fifty years, Social Security reform constituted the "third rail" of American politics. By the year 2000, however, high-level worries about aging boomers' impact upon entitlements were penetrating public discussion via a series of books, beginning with Peter Peterson's grim projections in *Gray Dawn* (1999) and a later book *Running on Empty* (2004). Other examinations of pending demographic-economic crises include Laurence J. Kotlikoff and Scott Burns's *The Coming Generational Storm* (2004), Alice M. Rivlin and Joseph Antos's *Restoring Fiscal Sanity*

(2007), James Schulz and Robert Binstock's *Aging Nation* (2006), and Andrew L. Yarrow's *Forgive Us Our Debts* (2008).[18]

Thus, when Kathleen Case-Kirschling became the first baby boomer eligible to apply for Social Security on October 15, 2007, in a special ceremony at the Washington Press Club, the event was portrayed with gallows humor by the *Washington Post's* Dana Milbank: "When it comes to the nation's finances, Kathleen Casey-Kirschling is Public Enemy No. 1. Her offense: being born. Specifically, being born on Jan. 1, 1946, just a tick after midnight. That made her the first member of the 80 million-strong baby-boom generation, which, starting next year will begin to bankrupt the nation by crashing the Medicare and Social Security systems. . . . As the boomers retire, Social Security will go into the red in 2017 and become insolvent 24 years later, according to the system's trustees. Medicare, meanwhile, starts bleeding in 2013 and goes under in 2019."[19]

Milbank joined his fellow *Post* columnists George Will, David Broder, and Paul Samuelson, along with the former Office of Management and Budget director David Walker (now with the Peter G. Peterson Foundation), as among the most publicly visible members of a "doomsday chorus" of policy thinkers forecasting that aging boomers would bankrupt Medicare and Social Security. This gloomy policy choir gained converts and grew louder in the wake of the 2008 economic crises. The fiscal future of Social Security has become too important to ignore.

Boomers may be as dependent as their parents have been upon Social Security and Medicare. This is largely because aging boomers' other forms of retirement savings are far more vulnerable to stock market and real estate fluctuations. Boomers have borne the brunt of a social policy revolution that the political scientist Jacob Hacker terms a "Great Risk Shift."[20] The risks and costs of retirement and health care policies have been shifted from institutions—especially employers—to individuals.

Corporations that once provided relatively generous lifetime retirement pensions ("defined benefit plans") and inexpensive health insurance are shifting costs and responsibilities onto employees. Traditional pensions are being replaced by individual 401(k) retirement accounts ("defined-contribution pensions"). Health insurance policies have also moved toward higher employee monthly premiums and deductibles along with tightly regulated health maintenance organizations. As globalization has waxed, job security and institutional loyalty have dramatically waned.

The deep recession, stock market crash, and plummeting values in residential real estate have exposed the flaws in relying upon individual retirement accounts to replace traditional pensions. "'The 401(k) system has had a chance, and in my view, it has failed,'" declared Alicia Munnell, one of the nation's foremost retirement economics specialists.[21] (Recent stock market rebounds have temporarily quieted calls for major overhaul—but the need to reduce risk remains.)

The boomer age wave will also encounter several sociological crises. Aging boomers will have a diminished social support network compared to previous generations. Family forms that once cushioned old age have been weakened by high divorce rates, geographical dispersion, and relatively low boomer birthrates. And the most secularized generation in history will soon confront end-of-life crises in purpose and meaning that may be (or may not be) channeled into civic, religious— or political—activity. These changes will intensify boomers' old-age anxieties.

Changing Demographics

Boomers' senior power potential will depend not only upon developments within their generation but also upon powerful external changes shaping both boomers and American society. Younger Americans who will be asked to subsidize aging baby boomers' entitlements differ profoundly from their elders not only in terms of age but in terms of ethnic and cultural characteristics as well.

The boomer-driven age wave coincides with a second demographic revolution produced by large-scale immigration and globalization of markets, customers, and workers. The latter is challenging the twentieth-century institutions that nurtured many young and maturing white, middle-class boomers: traditional "Ozzie and Harriet" families, broad support for public schools, civic associations, long-term employer-employee relationships, and strong identification with the nation-state.[22] These arrangements underpinned the social contract and the intergenerational trust and transfer payments built into Social Security and Medicare.

The immigration of large numbers of poor people into a postindustrial nation undergoing major economic changes poses the question of whether the nation may become divided between an older, relatively wealthy and well-educated white boomer gerontocracy and a younger, poorer, less educated, more ethnically diverse "Global America." Mass immigration is rapidly changing the demographic landscape. More than 75 percent of boomers are white, and they grew up during a period of relative ethnic homogeneity and economic prosperity in American history. A major study by the Harvard political scientist Robert Putnam suggests that immigration-driven ethnic diversity reduces civic participation, social solidarity, and the spirit of *E Pluribus Unum*—at least in the short term.[23]

Whites are now a demographic minority in large diverse states such as California, Texas, and New York. Nationwide, a majority of high school students are "of color."[24] But whites still constitute a large political majority. As Peter Schrag has argued in *California: America's High-Stakes Experiment,* whites in that bellwether state have locked in their dominant status by restricting new taxes and state government expenditures via a series of successful ballot propositions.[25] By 2010, these demographic strains and legal strictures combined to produce political gridlock, the largest state deficit in American history, and the unheard-of possibility of a state declaring "bankruptcy."

The prospect of California-style divisions spreading into the rest of the nation has led scholars at the New America Foundation, and also the University of Southern California policy scholar Dowell Myers (author of *Immigrants and Boomers*), to propose a new social contract for a changing America.[26] A new report by Brookings Institution scholars emphasizes the need to manage "an impending national transformation."[27]

Indeed, the nation's corporate and political leaders (including those at AARP) have been increasingly worried about the emergence of a fractured, two-tiered society in which a disproportionately white, well-educated, and well-off boomer gerontocracy battles to maintain old-age entitlements against an increasingly younger, multiethnic, multicultural generation that desires more public resources for middle-aged parents and children.

The desire to renew and expand the nation's social contract clearly underpinned the narrowly successful passage of major health care reform in March 2010. And it is likely to be more explicitly articulated in Social Security and Medicare reforms that are sure to follow. AARP has been a major voice in these efforts, especially through its massive "Divided We Fail" campaign, an AARP-headed alliance with the Business Roundtable, the Service Employees International Union, and the National Federation of Independent Businesses. Indeed, the campaign's goals of promoting "affordable, quality health care for all Americans" were directly echoed in the title of the final legislation: the Patient Protection and Affordable Care Act. (AARP has since taken a leading role in defending the legislation to members and the general public.)

While AARP has been anticipating changing demographics and the need for a renewed social contract, its immediate survival still depends upon its ability to recruit *and retain* a critical mass of aging boomer members. AARP wants to win that generation's hearts and minds, their money and trust. But though the organization has studied aging boomers more extensively than anyone else, even AARP's researchers admit they still have much to learn.

PLAN OF THE BOOK

Who are the boomers—especially the Older Boomers? The next chapter takes up these questions, mapping boomers' shared history, their distinctive cultural traits, and their current demographics—with an overview on economic inequalities and lifestyle issues. Chapter 2 opens with a discussion of the changing economic environment wrought by "supercapitalism" and demographic change, the advent of the "risk shift" from institutions to individuals in matters of retirement savings and health care, and a brief look at boomers' retirement risks before the economic storms of 2008. The interplay of aging boomers and younger immigrant populations is examined with special reference to the nation's demographic laboratory, California, America's Tomorrowland, where a "Sociological San Andreas Fault Line" illustrates the coalescing divisions of age, race, and class.

Chapter 3 focuses on the relationship of age and politics and boomers' senior power potential. There are questions as to whether the presumed "senior bloc" has been a reality or more of a myth. I examine the factors that might favor or inhibit the political mobilization of aging boomers. Of particular interest is whether they have sufficient generational cultural consensus and economic convergence of interests to become a voting bloc or active social movement. The latter is furthered by threatened reductions in Social Security and Medicare. But both cultural consensus and economic convergence have been fragmented by the emergence of a class/educational/cultural divide—as seen in the interplay of age, class, education, and race in boomers' participation and voting in the 2008 elections. While the surge in "youth power" that drove the Obama presidential campaign appears to have waned, aging boomers are ascendant postelection players in the Tea Party movement.

Chapter 4 turns to the financial and sociological impact of the real estate and stock market meltdowns as well as the so-called Great Recession. The depth and breadth of these crises severely tested boomers' characteristic optimistic, individualistic response to problems.

Boomers' political response to such issues in the 2008 presidential election illustrated the class/educational/cultural divide outlined in chapter 3. The election also intensified negative stereotyping of boomers—much of it by boomers themselves. Stereotyping tended to follow class-cultural lines: first, the upscale stereotype of boomers as greedy, irresponsible yuppies who didn't save for retirement, and second, the downscale stereotype of white, small-town, middle- and working-class boomers as hyperpatriotic, religious, racist reactionaries opposed to immigration, ethnic diversity, and change. Neither stereotype garners much empathy or sympathy, and both could politically undercut boomers in the coming debates over Medicare and Social Security reforms.

Chapter 5 focuses upon the largely unstudied transformation of the nation's largest senior citizen lobby, AARP. This forty-million-member organization has been changing to adapt more readily to rapidly changing economic and demographic realities. In trying to shed its "greedy geezer" stereotype and become the nation's preeminent agent of social change and arbiter of generational equity, AARP is attempting to recruit and retain aging boomer members while also seeking to broaden its generational and ethnic base in pursuit of its mission to promote positive change for "everyone who has a birthday."

Chapter 6 opens with a look at AARP's fiftieth-anniversary celebration and then turns to the political and policy dilemmas faced by the organization in trying to balance its "trust" and "warrior" brands in supporting (and now defending) the narrowly successful Democratic health care reform legislation, the Patient Protection and Affordable Care Act.

Chapter 7 explores aging boomers' political future in terms of the choices of "Me, We, or AARP?" I return to chapter 3's themes of tension between boomers' optimistic individualism and their increasing awareness of economic vulnerability, as well as the growing class and ideological gap between elites and large segments of the middle and working classes that divides both boomers and other Americans. I also focus upon waning national identity and declining levels of interpersonal and institutional trust—perilous contexts in which serious proposals for Social Security and Medicare reforms are just beginning to be made.

As I have observed repeatedly at many professional conferences: "No one knows boomers like AARP." Indeed, they must.

AARP is positioning itself to be a primary arbiter of generational politics, embattled entitlement policies, and health care reform and to channel any surge of boomer-based political power. And unless aging boomers get their act together and mobilize on their own, AARP is likely to become "leader of the pack" (to use the title of a 1960s rock ballad). How successful AARP is at brokering boomers' endangered entitlements while balancing the needs of future members will be a major sociological story during the second decade of the twenty-first century.

CHAPTER ONE

Boomer Basics

Generation, Culture, Demographics

> For here is the easy question: can a generation—reared
> in affluence, schooled in self-importance, comparatively
> ignorant of national sacrifice—admit that the country can't
> support it as grandly in its old age as it did in its youth?
> —Howard J. Fineman (2006)

In the pre-2008 glow of prosperity and optimism, the buzz at the 2007 Fourth Annual "What's Next? Boomer Business Summit" in Chicago was that business and corporate America were finally rediscovering the vast baby boomer market. Advertisers and marketers once studied and catered to the huge numbers of baby boomer children and adolescents. Corporate America's first generational mass marketing effort in the 1950s had given the boomers much of their identity and culture via television and rock music. But as middle-aged boomers became so much more diverse in economic status and lifestyles, interest in generation-focused research waned. No more.

"Welcome to the revolution," AARP's chief brand officer Emilio Pardo told the three hundred registered conference attendees. More diverse and powerful than any previous generation, "boomers have transformed every life stage through which they've moved. Boomers want to feel good, look good, are still creative and idealistic. They want choices, have a voice (in national affairs), and they have 'attitude.'"

However, warned Pardo, boomers resent being stereotyped and approached only on the basis of age. "Focus on needs and make the individual connection," he told the audience. AARP had found that boomers' main concerns were financial security, health, community, the need to contribute and leave a legacy, and "play" (through leisure and recreation).

Mary Furlong, the prime mover behind the boomer business summits and author of *Turning Silver into Gold*, insisted that the aging boomer market could not be ignored.[1] "There is no market opportunity larger than the boomers," the Santa Clara University business professor told the conference. But marketing to boomers meant understanding the trends shaping their needs and wants: global markets, longevity, life stage transitions ("e-shocks" such as divorce or death of a loved one), technology, and spirituality. Boomers constituted a pot of gold for businesses in health, housing, travel, networking, and services. And busy boomers, seeking second careers and new life purposes, might propel an explosion in small business growth.[2]

Indeed, many audience members seemed to be women over age fifty who were in some sort of career transition—unemployed, marginally employed, or trying to start new careers. (Approximately two-thirds of the audience and speakers were women.) Corporate America was conspicuous by its relative absence. AARP was very much the primary sponsor and supplied several major speakers. Very few conference speakers and panelists were from major corporations. Intel, Phillips, Verizon, Microsoft, and Walmart were listed as minor sponsors.

Other boomer-business conferences reportedly failed to register much increased interest or participation from corporate America even before the Great Recession dampened enthusiasm—and budgets—for expanding market frontiers. Jennifer Mann, a *Kansas City Star* reporter, was puzzled by this neglect. The one hundred million consumers over age fifty control eight trillion dollars in assets, more than 70 percent of disposable dollars, "yet they barely get passing notice from American advertisers." A major reason, marketing experts informed her, is that "a big problem in the ad agency world is that so many employees of agencies, particularly those who work on the creative side, are mostly in their 20s and 30s. Either they have no interest in working on campaigns targeted to older people, or they don't know how to."[3]

Nonetheless, through their sheer numbers, the boomer age wave is becoming a mass market inevitability. There has been an obvious surge of television and print media advertising toward boomers in the marketing realms noted by AARP's Emilio Pardo: health-related products (from Viagra to Flow-Max to Cancer Care Centers), financial planning (the rock-and-roll advertisements of both Fidelity and Ameriprise Financial Services), and leisure and recreation. In the realm of "political marketing," strategists in the 2008 presidential campaigns quickly realized that age had become a key voting behavior variable during the Democratic primary contest between boomer Hillary Clinton and self-advertised "postboomer" Barack Obama. Voters under thirty heavily favored Obama; those over age fifty—especially working-class women—generally favored Clinton. In the subsequent general election against John McCain, Obama won the under-thirty vote by 2–1.

In this chapter I am primarily interested in defining the key concept of generation and in outlining the basic cultural and demographic characteristics of baby boomers, especially the Older Boomers (born 1946–55). I will begin addressing questions that will recur throughout the book: Who are the boomers? What are their similarities? What are their differences? How have they changed? What are their needs, hopes, fears?

Boomers' culture and demographics will strongly influence a broader question: Will they have sufficient cultural cohesion and economic and sociological convergence to politically mobilize? Or will their intense individualism, coupled with inequalities and other demographic differences, forever fragment them? And, if so, will AARP become their leader by default?

BOOMER SELF-IDENTIFICATION

A vital preliminary question for marketers, political analysts, and social scientists is: Do boomers think of themselves as boomers? And do common generational experiences provide a *lasting* basis for shared perceptions on economics, politics, culture, and other realms?

Currently, boomer self-identification seems superficial at best. A recent survey by Boomer Insights Generation Group (a subunit of the huge Edelman marketing and public relations firm) finds that 71 percent of boomers identify themselves as such, but fully 28 percent do not.[4] The latter are mostly Younger Boomers. A MetLife Mature Market Institute survey discovered that the oldest boomers were more likely to favor the label than the youngest. Eighty-three percent of the "Oldest Boomers" (born in 1946) liked the term or liked it somewhat, but nearly half of the Youngest Boomers (born in 1964) indicated that they didn't like the term, and another 20 percent indicated that they didn't know whether they liked it or not.[5] Overall, though, a 2008 Harris Interactive poll found that boomers were more satisfied with their generational label than other age groups.[6]

The chief impediment to boomer generational self-identification is their fierce individualism—a hallmark trait found in nearly all research on boomers. Boomers' individualism is also a headache for marketers and advertisers.

"Boomers refuse to be identified as part of a group," former *AARP Magazine* editor Steve Slon told me. They don't "feel part of the same tribe."[7] He should know. ARRP tried to market a monthly magazine specifically for boomer members titled *My Generation*. It failed. (*AARP Magazine* is now quietly segmented by subscribers' age groups: fifties, sixties, and seventy or above.) "Please Don't Call Us That!" was the title of Joe Queenan's 2010 protest against the "baby boomer" label published on the AARP Web site.[8]

Boomers' sensitivity to collective categorization forces marketers to group "the aging generation into categories that give the illusion of individuality, they hope, while still encompassing millions of people," observed the *New York Times* reporter Charles Duhigg.[9] Contemporary boomer-focused advertising sometimes gently references "generation" but never the word *boomer.*

Boomers' lack of active generational identification has led to disappointments for Web site founders hoping to attract boomers as boomers. Eons.com is the prime example. Launched in 2005 with great fanfare by Jeff Taylor, founder of the successful Monster.com jobs Web site, Eons. com has narrowed its original broadly based focus on "living life on the flip side of 50." The broader, more commercial and information-based mission (including an obituary page) has been dropped. Eons.com now operates primarily as a "friendship engine" for middle-aged people who want to meet others with similar interests via a wide range of affinity groups.[10] Many other boomer Web sites are relationship oriented or, like Baby Boomer Headquarters.com, focused upon cultural nostalgia. Boomer-oriented Web sites come and go.[11]

But boomers' collective consumer profile is nonetheless being mapped by entrepreneurs and corporations who track the Web sites boomers most frequently visit. (Again, as AARP's Pardo noted, these are in the areas of finance, health, news, and recreation—though he did not publicly admit that for boomer men the latter includes both sports and pornography.)

Boomers likely will become much more age conscious as they cross various age thresholds, including "senior citizen discounts" (as low as age fifty), voluntary or forced retirement, and eligibility for Social Security (for reduced benefits at age sixty-two) and Medicare (age sixty-five). Most especially, boomers will acquire collective consciousness via intimations of mortality as they confront early indicators or the actual onset of chronic disease. (Cancer patient Diana Wagman was surprised to discover how many of her age forty- and fifty-something friends smoked marijuana. The reasons: pain—"We're all beginning to fall apart . . . a couple of tokes really take the edge off the sciatica, rotator cuff injuries, irritable bowel syndrome, and migraine"; and anxiety—"to relax, to forget our disappointing careers and mask our terror of not just our own future but the future of our kids as well.")[12]

As AARP's savvy marketers have discovered, one broad basis of unity for Older Boomers is the music and television of their youth. Older Boomers came of age during an era that was unusually ethnically and culturally homogeneous. They were more uniformly molded than previous generations by postwar prosperity, suburbanization, television—and especially a youth-based commercial music industry. "They were the 'Golden Kids,' the first automobile-centered, 'transistor teens,' the focus of the radio music industry," said Marc Fisher, *Washington Post* columnist and author of *Something in the Air*. "They are the first generation to think of themselves as such."[13]

But demographic differences within this huge age cohort make it difficult for boomers—or others—to see anything like a unified group. AARP's marketers are still studying the wide range of economic, educational, ethnic, and other differences among boomers. "More than ever, we realize boomers are a large and diverse generation," AARP's savvy former CEO Bill Novelli told me. "We have to do a lot of segmentation research."[14]

Again: Who are the baby boomers, especially those Older Boomers born from 1946 to 1955? And what, exactly, *is* a generation?

KARL MANNHEIM'S CONCEPT OF GENERATIONS

No one has better defined and explained the term *generation* than the German sociologist Karl Mannheim in his classic 1923 essay "The Problem of Generations."[15] Mannheim located the study of generations within the wider enterprise of the sociology of knowledge: how individuals and groups come to "know what they know" through shared experiences and interpretations of events and processes within specific historical and sociocultural contexts.

Mannheim likened the concept of generation to the more popular Marxian concept of social class—a category of people who share similar economic or occupational positions. Just as an economic class can become an organized, active "class-conscious" group, so, too, can a generation. A generation shares the same historical location. They collectively experience and interpret the key events of that period. Many will think and respond to their shared passage in the same way. Distinctive generational identities may arise. They may begin to think and act as a group.

The concept of generation is often blurred with the related concepts of age cohort, period effects, and cohort effects. An "age cohort" is simply an inert demographic category. For example, the baby boom is usually defined as those born between 1946 and 1964. But as discussion inevitably turns to boomers' social history and generational identity, that broad category is usually subdivided into two "minicohorts," which I identify throughout this book as Older Boomers (born 1946–55) and Younger Boomers (born 1956–62). "Period effects" are events or processes during a particular historical time frame that affect all groups. For example, World War II affected most Americans in the 1940s; in the 1950s, the increased availability of television was a major information and entertainment transformation. An "age cohort effect" is the impact of such events on a particular age group during a particular life stage. For instance, men of military draft age were most directly affected by World War II; baby boomers "grew up" on television in the 1950s.[16]

The gerontologist Robert Binstock has illustrated how age cohort and period effects interacted in shaping older voters' behavior in the 2008 elections. A majority of voters over sixty-five picked the Republican presidential candidate John McCain John McCain over Obama (53 to 45 percent). But Binstock demonstrates that the vote for McCain was particularly strong among voters age sixty-five to seventy-four, the "Eisenhower cohort" of older voters, who in their youth were strongly shaped by the 1950s presidency of Dwight Eisenhower. This political cohort has manifested these GOP-leaning "period effects" throughout their voting history.[17]

Mannheim maintained that, though an age cohort may obtain consciousness of itself as a generation, the salience of generational consciousness varies. Some generations may have a strong sense of collective consciousness; others may not. "The drama of youth" shapes each generation's shared perspective as they make "potentially fresh contact with current events and 'present problems.'"[18] But subgroups or "generational units" may also encounter and interpret the same historical processes differently. For example, boomer subgroups differently interpreted the 1960s and its liberal legacy—resulting in the long-running "culture wars" that postboomer President Obama promised to transcend.

AMERICA'S GENERATIONAL LANDSCAPE

Throughout the book, I shall refer to five generational classifications drawn from studies by both the Pew Research Center and the Metlife Mature Market Institute:[19]

- *The Greatest Generation:* approximately 8 million people over age eighty-four (born 1910–27), who were molded as young adults by enduring the Great Depression and by fighting and winning World War II. They have been famously lionized by Ronald Reagan as the generation that "saved the world."
- *The Silent Generation:* an estimated 31.5 million people aged sixty-six to eighty-three (born 1928–45), who had their childhood and adolescence shaped by the Great Depression and World War II and who moved into adulthood during the general era of conformity and prosperity in the postwar years.
- *Baby Boomers:* 78 million people aged forty-seven to sixty-five (born 1946–64), defined by a nineteen-year postwar spike in the

birthrate. The Older Boomers were raised with high expectations during the prosperous 1950s and 1960s but were shaped by conflict and division over civil rights and the Vietnam War and also by several memorable historical events, ranging from the assassination of John F. Kennedy in 1963 to the Watergate scandal and resignation of Richard Nixon in the early 1970s; Younger Boomers came of age in the aftermath of all this and were shaped by the increasing educational and occupational changes wrought by globalization.

· *Generation X:* 49.6 million people aged thirty-five to forty-six (born 1965–76), also called the "Baby Bust," who had to cope with changing institutional structures and have become defined by their entrepreneurial, savvy skills.

· *Gen Y or "the Millennial Generation":* 76.5 million people aged seventeen to thirty-four (born 1977–94), who came of age in the twenty-first century. Nearly as large as the boomer generation, they are seen as very technologically savvy and as the most politically liberal—they were viewed as the backbone of Barack Obama's presidential campaign.

Generational identities are not strong but may be growing. When the Pew Research Center asked respondents from all adult age groups what made their own generation distinctive or "unique," the top choice of traits among the competitive boomers was, not surprisingly, "work ethic"; somewhat more surprisingly, the generation with the 1960s rebellious stereotype also viewed itself as "respectful." And a small percentage of boomers identified themselves as "baby boomers"—the only group to self-identify as a generation. Three of the four age groups cited "work ethic" as a key characteristic; Gen X and Millennials cited "technology use" (table 1). But these lists of cultural traits only begin to suggest the complexity of an identifiable, basic shared culture and ideology among baby boomers—one that has remained fairly consistent over time.

TABLE I

What Makes Your Generation Unique?

Millennial	Gen X	Boomer	Silent
Technology use (24%)	Technology use (12%)	Work ethic (17%)	World War II, Depression (14%)
Music/pop culture (11%)	Work ethic (11%)	Respectful (14%)	Smarter (13%)
Liberal/tolerant (7%)	Conservative trad'l (7%)	Values/morals (8%)	Honest (12%)
Smarter (6%)	Smarter (6%)	"Baby boomers" (6%)	Work ethic (10%)
Clothes (5%)	Respectful (5%)	Smarter (5%)	Values/morals (10%)

SOURCE: *Millennials: Confident. Connected. Open to Change* (Washington, DC: Pew Research Center, February, 2010), 5.

NOTE: Based on respondents who said their generation was unique/distinct. Items represent individual, open-ended responses. Top five responses are shown for each age group. Sample sizes for subgroups are as follows: Millennials, n = 527; Gen X, n = 173; Boomers, n = 283; Silent, n = 205.

BOOMER CULTURE AND IDEOLOGY

A strong consensus in the growing literature on baby boomers is that their childhood and adolescent experiences forged a shared, though very general, sociological identity, especially among those who were suburban, white, and middle or upper middle class.[20] The 1946–64 baby boom resulted from (1) the postponement of childbearing by older women during the Depression and World War II, (2) a three-year drop in women's average age of first childbirth, and (3) an overall rise in the number of births. The boom was sustained by unusually favorable economic and cultural trends. The long period of postwar economic prosperity and the suburban housing boom encouraged a large number of babies. Family life was idealized, children and marriage were celebrated, and a powerful, popular "procreation ethic" took hold during the longest economic expansion in U.S. history. In this environment "contraceptive vigilance could be relaxed because penalties for not doing so were not so harsh."[21]

"Many a child's life did indeed match the *Happy Days* image.... The future looked happy and uncomplicated like the *Jetsons*," observe *Generations* coauthors William Strauss and Neil Howe.[22] Indeed, nearly 80 percent of boomers report being raised in "Ozzie and Harriet" two-parent households—in contrast to the 61 percent figure for today's twenty-something Millennials.[23]

The sociologist Paul Light agrees that boomers were raised in a prosperous era that encouraged value change, tolerance, and rejection of traditional social roles; they internalized optimism and great expectations forged by television and Madison Avenue. But Light emphasizes that competitive economic and social crowding fostered individualism and detachment from institutions. Indeed, Boomers' notorious focus on the self was inevitable, a "generational sensibility rooted in numbers and mindset—boomers could not have turned out any other way," conclude Yankelovich researchers Walker Smith and Ann Clurman.[24]

The stereotype of adolescent and young adult boomers as widely involved in radical politics and the hedonistic counterculture is just that. Strauss and Howe point out that political radicals and "hippies" represented only 10 to 15 percent of boomers; many boomers' opposition to the Vietnam War was motivated more by their aversion to the military draft.[25] (Hollywood producer Steven Spielberg admitted as much to a *Rolling Stone* reporter: "I was obsessed with staying out of Vietnam. . . . My immediate political activity was based on self-preservation.")[26]

Indeed, even the most idealistic of the nineteen influential boomer change agents studied by Michael Gross became more pragmatic as they moved into middle age. "The counter-culturalists' revolutionary pipe dreams have been overturned or co-opted. . . . Like First Baby

Boomer Bill Clinton we are not so much committed moralists as morally flexible, ambition-driven pragmatists far more like the parents we rebelled against than we may care to admit."[27]

Yet boomers' youthful idealism and social movement participation yielded lasting, positive changes. *Greater Generation* author Leonard Steinhorn correctly argues that the 1960s liberation movements, especially feminism and the civil rights movement, permanently changed boomers and society.[28] The historian Steve Gillon also credits the importance of feminism in changing society, especially by propelling boomer women into the workplace and by providing new models for movement building and political networking.[29]

But the 1960s social movements and resultant changes also polarized boomers and other Americans—a split played out for nearly four decades of "culture wars." This dueling liberal-conservative boomer political heritage was epitomized in the vastly different political personas of the first two boomer presidents, Bill Clinton and George W. Bush. Gillon sees boomers as a "generation at war with itself," agreeing with earlier observations by *Generations* authors William Strauss and Neil Howe that the culture wars reflect class, religious, and geographical divides.[30]

Strauss and Howe flatly reject the notion of self-interested aging boomer politics. An intensely idealistic and moralistic generation, boomers, with their zeal for social reform and the greater good, will ultimately transcend their self-centered individualism and the specter of age-based politics. However, as we shall see in chapter 3, the sometimes militant idealism and reformism of boomers in their youth was largely the ideology of the educated, evolving professional and managerial boomer upper middle class. Those further down the economic ladder faced increasingly competitive labor markets in which idealism quickly gave way to pragmatic realism regarding rising economic instability and survival in a world dominated by global supercapitalism.

BOOMERS IN MIDLIFE: INDIVIDUALISTIC, OPTIMISTIC, AND "FOREVER YOUNG"

Beginning in the 1970s, increasingly competitive job markets changed college students' educational and career choices. Men, especially, were forced to become more practical. As Landon Jones noted, "In the sixties, students studied sociology so they could change the world; in the seventies they studied psychology so they could change themselves; in the eighties they will study business administration so they can survive."[31]

The journalist Tom Wolfe skewered upper-middle-class middle-aged boomers as the self-obsessed, self-indulgent "Me Generation."[32] But the social scientist Paul Light detailed a somewhat darker boomer ethos: a work-driven rugged individualism detached from civic society and mistrustful of government. He saw middle-aged boomers as motivated by quests for (1) individual economic opportunity and (2) personal meaning and safety. Boomers became mistrustful of large institutions and developed little long-term loyalty. They tried to find a philosophy of life in their work—often at the expense of personal life and civic participation.[33] Their intense individualism and self-reliance bred an unforgiving outlook. "More than any other generation, Boomers blame failure on the individual. . . . They feel in control of their financial lives."[34] Light detected an ideological drift toward "political and social survivalism" and a proclivity for privatization of public problems.[35] (Ten years later, the Harvard political scientist Robert Putnam, in his classic book *Bowling Alone,* marshaled survey research data to confirm suspected trends in boomers' declining civic involvement.)[36]

As the twenty-first century dawned, AARP's "Boomers at Midlife" survey and focus group data (2002, 2004) found that middle-aged boomers remained resilient, optimistic individualists with a can-do ideology that attributed individual success—or lack thereof—to personal factors such as motivation, confidence, or willpower. One in three respondents stated that "nothing" was keeping them from achieving their goals. Nearly two-thirds of older boomers (64 percent) and three-fourths of younger boomers (73 percent) strongly agreed with the statement "What happens to me in the future mostly depends on me"—even though fewer than half perceived "a great deal" of personal control over future personal finances, physical health, or work or career. Nearly 60 percent remained confident that they were "very likely" to achieve work/career goals, while another 53 percent thought they would reach financial goals.[37]

In their 2007 book *Generation Ageless,* Yankelovich researchers Smith and Clurman identified three universal boomer traits: (1) youthfulness, (2) impact—the desire to have influence and make a difference, and (3) belief in personal development through empowerment and continuous progression.[38] Like other researchers, they described boomers as individualistic innovators and rule breakers who emphasized control and choice and who were flexible and comfortable with change. Attitudes toward government were characteristically guarded: 80.5 percent agreed that "government isn't the best answer for most of the problems we face." (Yet a paradox: nearly 70 percent agreed that people had the right to "the best medical care.") Boomers still didn't believe much in the system and thought it might have to be reformed from the "outside." And they might be the ones to do it because "aging boomers have a lot of fight left in them."[39]

DEMOGRAPHICS, INEQUALITY, AND LIFESTYLE GROUPS

In 2010, Metlife Mature Market Institute completed an analysis of Older Boomers (born 1946–51), Middle Boomers (born 1952–58), and Younger Boomers (born 1959–64). The characteristics of these three subgroups are portrayed in table 2.

Generally speaking, occupational and educational changes are most evident among men in these three boomer subgroups. Older

TABLE 2

Characteristics of Major Boomer Subgroups

	Older Boomers (1946–51)		Middle Boomers (1952–58)		Younger Boomers (1959–64)	
Number (millions)	20,491,763		29,089,514		27,403,993	
Percent of boomer population	27%		38%		36%	
Percent of total population	7%		10%		9%	
Age in 2011	60–65		53–59		47–52	
Ethnic Composition (2009)						
Non-Hispanic white alone	76%		73%		69%	
Non-Hispanic black alone	10%		11%		12%	
Non-Hispanic Asian alone	4%		4%		4%	
All other races	2%		2%		2%	
Hispanic (any race)	8%		10%		13%	
Income by Household Type	Mean	Median	Mean	Median	Mean	Median
Married-couple families	$94,449	$73,255	$108,910	$86,657	$109,134	$88,184
Male householders living alone	$39,301	$26,763	$45,577	$32,658	$50,846	$36,258
Female householders living alone	$36,992	$26,752	$39,976	$30,687	$39,086	$31,291
Overall male householders	$43,332	$29,741	$50,253	$38,750	$56,603	$40,844
Overall female householders	$39,746	$29,176	$43,726	$33,980	$43,104	$33,910

TABLE 2 (continued)

Educational Level	Male	Female	Male	Female	Male	Female
Master's degree or higher	15%	12%	12%	11%	10%	10%
Bachelor's degree	20%	18%	18%	18%	18%	20%
Some college	26%	27%	27%	30%	25%	30%
High school graduate	27%	33%	32%	30%	34%	31%
Less than high school	12%	11%	11%	11%	12%	10%

Occupation	Male	Female	Male	Female	Male	Female
Production, transportation, and material moving	17%	7%	19%	6%	19%	7%
Construction, extraction, and maintenance	15%	1%	18%	1%	19%	1%
Farming, fishing, and forestry	1%	0%	1%	0%	1%	0%
Sales and office	17%	34%	15%	32%	14%	31%
Service	10%	17%	10%	17%	11%	19%
Management, professional, and related	42%	42%	37%	44%	36%	42%

Marital Status	Male	Female	Male	Female	Male	Female
Married	75.3%	65.0%	70.4%	65.9%	65.5%	65.4%
Widowed	2.5%	9.0%	1.5%	4.7%	1.0%	2.7%
Divorced	12.8%	17.0%	14.8%	17.6%	14.3%	16.8%
Separated	1.9%	1.8%	2.5%	3.1%	2.5%	3.6%
Never married	7.5%	7.1%	10.7%	8.7%	16.7%	11.4%

SOURCE: Metlife Mature Market Institute, Demographic Generational Profiles, 2010, http://www.metlife.com/mmi/research/generational -profiles.html#introduction.

Boomer men are better educated and have a more upscale occupational profile and a more conventional marital status. Nearly 35 percent have a bachelor's degree or higher versus 30 percent of Middle Boomer men and 28 percent of Younger Boomer men. Forty-two percent of Older Boomer men are in management, professional, and related occupations compared to 37 percent of Middle Boomer men and 36 percent of Younger Boomer men; the latter are the most "blue collar," with 19 percent employed in "construction, extraction, and maintenance."

Evidence of cultural changes toward marriage is striking: 75 percent of the Older Boomer men are married versus only 70 percent of Middle Boomer men and 65 percent of Younger Boomer men; only 7.5 percent of Older Boomer men are "never married," but that figure more than doubles for Younger Boomer men to 16.7 percent.

Older Boomers are the smallest of the three groups, the "whitest" (76 percent non-Hispanic white), and, somewhat surprisingly, the lowest paid. But among the three subgroups what is most striking are gender differences. The portrait of Older Boomers was largely reinforced in a Metlife Institute study published a few months later of "Early Boomers" (aged fifty-five to sixty-four). The newer report focused upon how demographic characteristics might affect retirement prospects. The profile of Early Boomers suggested that they were likely to work longer because the oldest segment (aged sixty to sixty-four) had the highest male college graduation rates ever achieved (before or since): 37 percent. (Thirty percent of Early Boomer women had college degrees, but college graduation trends for women have risen steadily: thus women aged thirty to thirty-four have the highest graduation level of 38 percent.) Early Boomers' labor force participation is at an all-time high, despite the gloomy economy. This is probably because three-quarters of Early Boomer women and three-fifths of Early Boomer men were in more recession-proof white-collar jobs. This positive occupational tilt also explains relatively high incomes: fully 37 percent of Early Boomer married couples earned more than $100,000 per year; another 15 percent of married couples earned $75,000 to $100,000 and 20 percent earned $50,000 to $75,000.[40]

About two-thirds of these Early Boomers were estimated to be grandparents—and the effects of the Great Recession register in data that a rising number of them are raising, or helping to raise, their grandchildren. This, in turn, may be related to the finding that approximately one in four Early Boomer families had adult children at home. (For reasons that are unexplained, the "Early Boomers" in the newer report had 10 percent fewer married couples than the "Older Boomers" of the previous study. Only 56 percent of Early Boomers were married couples; 26 percent were women householders, and 18 percent were male householders.)[41]

Neither of the 2010 Metlife studies contained data on assets, net worth, or political attitudes. A benchmark study by Annamaria Lusardi and Olivia Mitchell, using data from the federal government's 2004 Health and Retirement Study, explored the important dimensions of inequality within boomer ranks. The median total net worth of Older Boomers (born 1946–53) was just $151,500. Subtract housing and any business assets and this figure dropped to a paltry $48,000. But for the top 10 percent asset levels were considerably higher, $888,010 and $536,700 respectively, and for the top 5 percent they were $1,327,000 and $903,600.[42]

A 2007 Metlife profile of a "typical" Older Boomer just turning sixty-two suggested a positive relationship between age and net worth: average annual income was $71,400 and their average household net worth (excluding home value) was $257,800. They were comfortable being identified as baby boomers and didn't think they would be "old" for another seventeen years. Twice as many were conservative as liberal.[43]

But the stock market crash and real estate recession have taken a toll on boomers' net worth. By 2009 the Center for Economic Policy and Research found that boomers' median net worth had fallen 45 to 50 percent; a partial recovery later that year led Moody's to recalculate this loss as closer to 25 percent.[44]

Boomer Inequalities

Social class is one of the most powerful factors shaping political behavior and the life course. Rising inequality of incomes and assets among boomers mirrors increasing economic polarization throughout the nation. Economic inequalities, in turn, are strongly structured by race, education, and family status. How these inequalities might affect ideological divisions and prospects of generational mobilization will be more closely analyzed in chapter 3. For now, it should be kept in mind that inequalities cut two ways. On the one hand, relatively wealthy boomers might be more insulated against adverse policy or social changes and less likely to engage in organized political response; conversely, a sizable, less fortunate, anxious "boomer proletariat" might constitute a vulnerable, potent base for political protest.

Economically, two dominant trends have defined the baby boom generation for the past thirty years. First, the large number of young boomer men flooding the labor force in the 1970s and 1980s depressed wages, creating a lifelong income decline relative to that of their fathers. The second trend was partly in response to the first: large numbers of boomer women went to work full time outside the home. *Birth Quake* author Diane Macunovich concluded that by the end of the twentieth century "the much heralded closing of the male-female wage gap has resulted largely from a lowering of male wages, rather than from a real rise in female wages."[45]

To achieve middle-class lifestyles, boomers postponed marriage, had fewer children, and became dependent on two incomes. The proliferation of two-income families led to what Elizabeth Warren and Amelia Tiagi term the "two-income trap." As family incomes rose, the costs of middle-class life (especially housing and education) escalated even faster, stretching budgets and raising bankruptcy rates. The advent of global markets produced greater swings in annual family incomes and enhanced the value of advanced degrees.[46]

In their classic 2004 study *The Lives and Times of Baby Boomers,* Mary Elizabeth Hughes and Angela M. O'Rand found sharp inequalities among boomers structured by race, marital status, and educational attainment. Boomers cohabited, delayed marriage, divorced, and remarried, developing a pattern of "serial monogamy" along with a variety of other family forms. In becoming the best-educated generation in history, they closed and even reversed gender gaps in education. Conversely, race and ethnic educational attainment gaps increased. (Among Early Baby Boomers, 25 percent of whites were college graduates, compared to 45 percent of U.S.-born Asians and about 15 percent of blacks and U.S.-born Hispanics.) The result: highly educated, white and Asian two-income, stable families pulled further away from others with less education, such as immigrant Hispanics and especially large numbers of black one-parent families.[47]

The Brookings Institution demographer William Frey updated and confirmed these trends in 2010. The sheer size of the tsunami, he noted, would magnify the boomers' distinctive social and demographic attributes, especially inequality. And, noting changes in family structure, Frey predicted that boomers' "higher rates of divorce and separation, lower rates of marriage and fewer children signal the potential for greater divisions in seniorhood between those who will live comfortably and those who will have fewer resources available to them."[48]

As we shall see in subsequent chapters, these wide economic variations in boomers' incomes, assets, education, and family status profoundly structure competing political and cultural worldviews that thus far have fragmented any potential boomer political cohesion. Indeed, income and education strongly affect perceptions of whether retirement will be "the Golden Years"—or something far less.

Income and Retirement Confidence

For most Americans, increased income, education, and occupational levels are generally associated with positive feelings about oneself and society, greater political awareness, and higher levels of civic and political participation. Two major studies of how boomers "envision retirement" with surprisingly similar findings on how economic status influences retirement perspectives were done before the 2008 economic turmoil: one by AARP and another by Merrill Lynch.[49]

A 2004 AARP "Boomers Envision Retirement" study (of a representative sample of 2,001 adults, aged thirty-eight to fifty-seven) sorted boomers into five groups. Thirty-two percent were "Self Reliants." They had the highest median household income ($82,000), the highest percentages in professional and white-collar occupations and with bachelor-or-above degrees (43 percent), and the highest percent married (84 percent) and white (83 percent). Self Reliants contributed to retirement accounts and were confident about their retirement years.

"Enthusiasts" were 14 percent of the sample. They were also 83 percent white and were second to the Self Reliants in terms of median income ($78,000), occupation, educational attainment (33 percent with undergraduate degrees or higher), and percent married (79 percent); and they were the most eager to retire completely from all work. "The Anxious" were 17 percent of the sample, third in terms of income ($60,000) and percent married (64 percent); they were similar to the Enthusiasts in terms of percent in white-collar occupations (34 percent) and college graduates (33 percent). The Anxious were nervous about retirement savings and were skeptical about retirement health care coverage and Social Security and Medicare reliability.

"Today's Traditionalists" were 22 percent of the sample. Their median household income was $52,000; 53 percent were in blue-collar jobs; 63 percent were married and 15 percent never-married or single; they had the highest percentage of African Americans at 19 percent and were the most confident about Social Security and Medicare. "The Strugglers," 15 percent of the respondents, had the lowest household income ($32,000), the highest percentage of single/never-married (16 percent) and the lowest percentage married (57 percent); 60 percent had blue-collar jobs; 57 percent were female (the highest percentage of all groups), and 17 percent were black (the second-highest percentage of all groups). Not unexpectedly, they had little saved for retirement and were the most pessimistic about it. (Significantly, the groups did not vary in terms of median age.)

Merrill Lynch's 2005 "New Retirement" telephone survey of 3,448 baby boomers found five similar subgroups with strong correlations between income, assets, and retirement outlook: "Wealth Builders" (20 percent of those interviewed, with an average income of $84,000), "Empowered Trailblazers" (18 percent, $83,000), "Anxious Idealists" (20 percent, $66,000), "Leisure Lifers" (13 percent, $64,000), and "Stretched and Stressed" (18 percent, $60,000).[50] In the Merrill Lynch survey, nearly half the respondents were self-confident and positive; only one-third of the AARP respondents were confident.

In both surveys, future health insurance affordability was a potent source of anxiety. Fifty-eight percent of the AARP respondents didn't expect employer contributions to their postretirement health insurance; 43 percent didn't expect Medicare to cover most of their medical needs. The Merrill Lynch survey uncovered an especially grim insecurity: more respondents feared lack of affordable health insurance (53 percent) than death (17 percent).[51]

The findings of these studies are probably still valid. Indeed, the Great Recession has likely reinforced these patterns. New research presented in chapter 4 suggests that those in the higher income brackets have been more likely to remain employed, have regained much of the value of their retirement portfolios, and have therefore probably remained more confident about their retirement futures. The most "anxious" middle groups have likely become more anxious. And low-income Americans have been most vulnerable to being forced into an early and uncomfortable retirement by unemployment.

In terms of this book's focus on whether aging boomers may respond politically to threatening economic and social changes, the AARP and Merrill Lynch studies suggest that boomers' readiness to identify with one another in a common political cause (via voting or social movements) will depend upon their resources, their confidence, and their fears. As the data presented in early this chapter suggest, boomers tend to be strongly individualistic and optimistic. This outlook has profoundly hindered their ability to recognize and cope with systematic economic and occupational changes that were well under way even before the Great Recession.

ENCOUNTERING EARLY RECESSION REALITIES

Studies of boomers' history and surveys about their attitudes and values tell us little about how boomers have actually negotiated the realities of aging—and the worst economic crisis since the 1930s. At the outset of what was to become known as the Great Recession, I interviewed several experts and consultants who were on the front lines of research or consulting with aging boomers, especially with regard to the workplace. (Later in the book, I will deal with boomers' reactions to the middle and late phases of the long, deep downturn.)

AARP's savvy brand officer Emilio Pardo noted boomers' abiding sense of optimism and opportunity. "Boomers think 'there's always one more tomorrow.'"[52] But many financial planners and career consultants put a much darker spin on boomers' hopes for tomorrow: denial.

SeasonedPro founder and career consultant Richard Katz found that boomers' emphasis on individual responsibility and blame was inhibiting their ability to seek needed counsel and advice. "There's a cultural stigma against seeking help," sighed Katz, who has worked extensively with university alumni groups. "It's not considered cool. . . . And it's a double stigma if you get help and then still can't get a job." This is especially true for men, he added.

Katz believes age discrimination in the workplace persists despite antidiscrimination laws and labor shortage forecasts. "Employers aren't willing to pay for baby boomers," he's concluded. "I've heard the forecasts of labor shortages and need to hire older workers. But I don't see it. Send them people over age thirty-five and they'll say, 'That's not what we're looking for.'" Katz admits that some older workers with engineering or highly specialized skills may fare better. But he grimly recalled a University of Houston career conference where 250 employers set up recruitment tables for new graduates, but only eighteen employers did so in the SeasonedPro section. Thus Katz had recently reoriented SeasonedPro to upwardly mobile career seekers in their thirties and forties. (I suggested he rename his company and Web site "Lightly SeasonedPro." We both laughed uneasily.)[53]

Carleen MacKay, an expert on mature workforces and coauthor of *Return of the Boomers,* thought boomers' sheer numbers made them different. She was less certain about their alleged commitment to individualism. Instead, what struck MacKay about these "Kennedy generation optimists" was that they were "pioneers in consumerism, debt, and materialism." Boomers, she stated, had a proclivity for instant gratification. They bought huge houses with the result that "the house owns them, not vice versa." She worried that too many boomers were "bad planners." They were totally unprepared for the economic dislocations that MacKay foresaw: waves of layoffs and pension problems—caused by the increasing devaluation of "overpriced" midlevel jobs via globalization and outsourcing—that were gradually eroding the status and security of middle-class jobs.

She was equally unimpressed with the foresight of boomers who still had job security and lifetime pensions. "When I asked a conference of California public employees in their forties and fifties how many would take early retirement, virtually all of them raised their hands," MacKay told me. "But most hadn't thought at all about what they'd do afterwards."[54]

The career transition consultant Andrew Johnson found that his generally upscale clientele in Southern California banking and real estate were adjusting to changing job markets through individualistic efforts of retraining and persistent job searches. Nevertheless, he saw occasional signs of a longing to return to New Deal–era government safety nets. Like many others interviewed for this book, he saw something of a backlash against information overload and the plethora of choices in health care and retirement planning. "People don't want to look out for themselves all the time. They accept the new changes, but they don't necessarily like them."[55]

Carleen MacKay offered a darker reason behind boomers' unease. "Many of them are surprised that they are maturing in an America that no longer wants them in the workplace."

CHAPTER TWO

Old Age in a New Society

In our politics and economy, in family life and religion—in
practically every sphere of our existence—the certainties of
the eighteenth and nineteenth centuries have disintegrated
or been destroyed and, at the same time, no new sanctions or
justifications for the new routines we live, and must live, have
taken hold. . . . There is no plan of life.
  —C. Wright Mills (1950)

The old institutions of democratic capitalism, and the negotiations that took place within them, are gone. But no new
institutions have emerged to replace them. We have no means
of balancing.
  —Robert Reich (2007)

The remarkably similar analyses above describe two wrenching transitions in American society in two different centuries. In his 1950 classic
White Collar, the sociologist C. Wright Mills described the transformation from a nineteenth-century America of small business, small towns,
and small farms into a twentieth-century, urbanized industrial nation-
state with a large new immigrant populations and an increasing international trade and military presence.[1] And at the dawn of the twenty-first
century, the policy analyst Robert Reich in *Supercapitalism* portrayed
the nation's current passage from an industrial nation state into a society where global "supercapitalism" maximizes consumer and investor
choice while eroding major industries, democratic processes, and civic

society.[2] And, once again, mass immigration is producing what Brookings Institution scholars term "an impending national transformation."[3]

The rise of transnational supercapitalism, coupled with the increased tempo of international travel and migration, strains nation-state sovereignty, regulatory authority, and the feelings of shared national purpose and community. The United States and its citizens now operate in what Fareed Zakaria famously defined as a "Post-American World," a new competitive international order "defined and directed from many places and by many people." As dozens of other nations rapidly expand economically, U.S. economic, political, and cultural influence wanes.[4]

Baby boomers and the nation's largest entitlement programs, Social Security and Medicare, remain the creations of a relatively prosperous twentieth-century nation-state. It was a national community with a strong sense of *E Pluribus Unum* and an intergenerational compact forged by the Great Depression, World War II, and a long cold war with communism. Will this "Old America," its civic cohesion and social contract, its old-age entitlements, and the core institutions boomers knew so well, survive in a "New America" characterized by globalization, supercapitalism, multiculturalism, and mass immigration?

"In the Old America," observed former Reagan presidential speechwriter Peggy Noonan, "love of country was natural. You breathed it in. You either loved it or knew you should. In the New America, love of country is a decision. It's one you make after weighing the pros and cons. What you breathe in is skepticism and a heightened appreciation of the global view."[5]

Aging boomers will grow old in a new society. The taken-for-granted economic, political, and cultural order is rapidly changing. And, as I will argue later in the chapter, in many ways, California resembles this new society. It is America's Tomorrowland.

National political and cultural touchstones are losing meaning and relevance. The average age of voters in 2008 was forty-four. Younger voters have only dim, history-book memories of the formative events of past generations: the Great Depression, World War II, the assassination of President John Kennedy and his brother Bobby, the Vietnam War, civil rights and women's liberation, the Watergate scandal, and Ronald Reagan's presidency.[6] And a new wave of younger congressional candidates is set to replace significant numbers of boomer and Silent Generation politicians. "Congress is in the midst of the most significant generational shift since 1974," observes the *Weekly Standard* reporter Mathew Continetti, who points out that the average age in the House of Representatives is forty-seven and the average age of senators is sixty-three—relatively old by historical standards.[7]

As discussed in the previous chapter, baby boomers lived much of their lives during America's mid-twentieth-century zenith as the world's dominant cultural, economic, and military superpower. It was a social order built upon a broad, inclusive value system that nourished political and civic participation and a welfare state with "safety net" programs. Production and consumption occurred primarily within national boundaries. Modern Western culture was built upon the rational spirit of the European enlightenment and a secular outlook in which state and religion became increasingly separated.[8] Postwar boomers were raised with a somewhat schizophrenic faith in and fear toward scientific and technological advancement. Some Older Boomers still remember the Walt Disney animated ode to atomic power, *Our Friend the Atom*. But more of them recall the infamous "duck and cover" air raid drills and the fear of nuclear holocaust in a bipolar world dominated by the United States and the Soviet Union.

The Middle East oil embargos of the early 1970s heralded the weakening of U.S. global economic hegemony and served notice of an evolving, interdependent global economy. Germany and Japan were emerging from postwar reconstruction, and their increasingly competitive auto and steel industries led to mass factory layoffs and the midwestern "Rust Belt." As Reich points out in *Supercapitalism*, American corporations utilized new technologies (giant cargo ships, sophisticated computer programs, telecommunications) to automate production or relocate it overseas. In the 1980s and 1990s job losses began moving up the occupational ladder as globalization, "reengineering," and automation promoted "right-sized" organizations.

In the new twenty-first-century global society, geographical borders, national identity, and sovereignty fade. Third World workers migrate legally and illegally into First World nations. Many members of the elite and professional classes have become globe-trotting "citizens of the world," managing rapidly changing international enterprises, living in many lands, and being constantly on the go. Place, local community, and extended family assume less importance. The cultural diffusion of birth control and feminism has replaced the 1950s idealized "Ozzie-and-Harriet" two-parent, single-earner family with falling birthrates and a multiplicity of family forms.[9] Today, two-thirds of all American households have no children in the home.[10]

Baby boomers witnessed and facilitated the arrival of postmodern society's 24/7 "global village." Computers, the Web, the Internet, cable television, and cell phones compress time and distance—and diminish specific locales. Print media yield to digital domains. This march of technological innovation has democratized knowledge and information. Anyone with access to the Internet and the Web can become self-educated in all manner of subjects.

Ironically, hyperindividualistic boomers who generally mistrust major institutions and demand choice and control over their own lives may have gotten more of all this than they ever wanted. The advent of supercapitalism and lengthening life spans have accelerated an institutional shift of risk and responsibility for health care, retirement, and financial planning from employers to employees—a trend that Jacob Hacker terms "the Great Risk Shift."[11] The increased insecurity and inequality inherent in the mass transition to do-it-yourself retirement accounts became evident in 2008 when a long housing recession was compounded by an autumn stock market meltdown and the worst recession since the 1930s.

During 2008, boomers on the brink of retirement lost on average approximately 20 percent of their individual retirement accounts. Some fared worse. Eventually, many would recoup their losses by persevering with monthly 401(k) contributions and via a 2009 market rebound. Nevertheless, the financial and psychological scars remain. How did retirement in America become more precarious and unpredictable?

THE ROAD TO RISK-SHIFT RETIREMENT

In mid-February 2007, Washington, D.C., was hit by one of its worst ice-and-snow storms in thirty years, on the night before AARP's board of directors gathered for their annual public policy meeting. In spite of closed airports and roads, however, all of the board members, CEO Bill Novelli and his management team, and most guests were on time. Several political notables addressed the group, including senators Hillary Clinton, Joe Biden, Gordon Smith, and Jeff Sessions and congressional Democratic leader Rahm Emanuel. Peter Orszag, the Congressional Budget Office director (and the future Obama White House budget director), spoke about "budget issues and reform." Yet the speaker who generated the liveliest response was Yale political scientist Jacob Hacker (who avoided iced-in airports by prudently taking the Metroliner train).

"Freedom to choose means freedom to lose," Hacker warned in opening a thirty-minute presentation drawn from his recent book *The Great Risk Shift*. The title named what Hacker viewed as the defining trend of America's postindustrial economy: a massive transfer of economic risk from corporations and government and onto "the fragile balance sheets of American families."[12] Economic security has declined in several realms: (1) jobs—no more long-term security and employer-employee loyalty; (2) two-income families are now a necessity for many Americans to maintain middle-class lifestyles—and even so, families are experiencing much more volatile income swings, divorce, and rising bankruptcy rates; (3) retirement—major employers are discontinuing defined-benefit, lifetime pensions and offloading risk and responsibility via individual retirement accounts; and (4) health care—employers are shifting rising deductibles and monthly premium costs to employees, shifting both costs and responsibility via individualized "health savings accounts," or simply dropping health care coverage altogether. The advent of a new "personal responsibility" ideology justified this policy revolution, enabling corporate and political leaders to avoid shielding American families from changes wrought by globalization.

An AARP board member disagreed with Hacker's contention that corporations competing in global markets had little choice in reducing benefits. "Globalization is letting corporations out of the social contract," she said. Hacker disagreed. He argued that American corporations still maintain a sense of national loyalty.

Had he been present, the public policy expert Robert Reich would have sided with the questioner. In the more Darwinian landscape of *Supercapitalism,* Reich argues that even the largest and best-paying corporations have been forced to join a relentless, competitive, globalized race to the bottom in search of cheap, unregulated foreign labor markets. This has produced a rich, low-cost bounty of goods, services, and economic opportunities benefiting consumers and investors—armed with computerized search engines to seek out the best deals. Alas, "Consumers get great deals because workers get shafted." Also shafted are civic society and the spirit of *E Pluribus Unum.* "Markets," explains Reich, "are hugely efficient at responding to individual desires, but quite bad at responding to goals we would like to achieve together."[13]

In 2008, a Minneapolis pharmacist gave voice to such changes during a PBS election forum. "All my customers sense there's something deeply wrong," he told a reporter. "There's a lost sense of community, a lost sense of confidence. No one cares about anyone else . . . we're just a bunch of individuals. And," he added, "if you don't look at this disparity of incomes we will become the richest Third World country in the world."[14]

Both Hacker and Reich acknowledged that a return to the New Deal era was improbable, but the two authors became very active in promoting national health care reform. Both were obviously aware of what the

classical economist Joseph Schumpeter described as unfettered capitalism's basic dynamic of "creative destruction." Indeed, throughout
most of the 1990s and well into the twenty-first century many Americans enjoyed the fruits of supercapitalism's creative and positive consequences. But few had any idea of how much havoc supercapitalism
could wreak upon retired and soon-to-retire Americans who trusted a
financial system they believed had tamed capitalism's notorious boom-
and-bust cycles.

I shall discuss the full impact of the 2007–9 Great Recession upon
boomers' retirement prospects in chapter 4. For now, it is simply worth
noting that by 2010 retirement and uninsured medical expenses topped
the list of financial concerns for all Americans in a Harris Interactive
poll.[15] This represents a sharp and welcome attitude adjustment for an
American workforce that was largely unaware of retirement and health
care needs during a previous, more prosperous era in which two-thirds
of aging boomers were financially ill prepared for retirement.

Headed for a Fall

"I don't understand why people aren't taking care of their older selves,"
declared an exasperated Matt Greenwald in the autumn of 2007. One
of the nation's leading retirement researchers, Greenwald, an aging
boomer himself, snorted that his generation's retirement philosophy
had become "Do the Right Thing—Later."[16]

Most boomers' retirement fates depend upon whether they participate in employer-sponsored pension plans and how safe and stable
those plans are. The extent of American workers' pension plan participation can be difficult to assess because of the use of different data sets
and reporting sources. Generally speaking, perhaps half of all private
sector workers participate in some sort of employer-sponsored retirement plan.[17]

There is also a growing gap in the types of pensions offered
to public-sector and private-sector workers. About 80 percent of

public-sector workers are covered by a traditional, professionally managed defined-benefit (lifetime payout) pension plan—as opposed to more risky, individually managed retirement accounts (401[k] or IRA).[18] As for private-sector workers, an Employee Benefit Research Institute study using data for 2005 found that 10 percent of private-sector workers had only a defined-benefit pension; 27 percent had both defined-benefit and defined-contribution pensions (the percentage with both rose with income); and 63 percent had only a defined-contribution 401(k)-type plan.[19] (The political implications of this private-versus-public "pension envy" will be discussed more fully in chapter 4.)

With specific regard to boomers, a 2006 Metlife survey of boomers turning sixty-two found that nearly half were covered by a defined-benefit plan; 50 percent had a 401(k) and 50 percent had an IRA.[20] The most optimistic finding was in a 2007 Fidelity Research Institute Retirement Index study: approximately 62 percent of preretirees aged fifty-five and above expected to receive a pension (through self or spouse), providing a median annual pension income stream of $21,106.[21]

Age and job tenure (number of years at the same job) are major sources of variations in 401(k) account savings. A precrash Employee Benefit Research Institute (EBRI) study found that, through 2006, boomers in their fifties had an average 401(k) balance of $148,927, ranging from $80,465 (for those on the job for five to ten years) to $192,003 (with twenty to thirty years on the job) . For those in their forties, 401(k) balances averaged $108,262 and ranged from $74,075 (for those on the job for five to ten years) to $146,489 (for those in their position from twenty or more years). The median account balance for boomers was approximately $111,000. (For all 401(k) savers, the average account balance was $121,202; the median amount was $66,650.)[22]

American workers are grossly unprepared for the Great Risk Shift. They tend to exhibit overconfidence, ignorance, and little policy awareness or preparation toward retirement planning and realities, according to an EBRI survey. They remain slow in understanding retirement system changes; are counting on retirement benefits that won't be there;

assume they have more long-term care insurance than they actually have; and know little about the eligibility age for full Social Security benefits.[23] (A Tiburon Strategic Advisors study found that 62 percent of American consumers expect to receive pensions when they retire; however, only 41 percent acknowledged that they or their spouses currently have such a pension.)[24]

Being married does not improve retirement planning readiness. A Fidelity Investments study found that only 38 percent of couples jointly discuss investment decisions for retirement savings; 44 percent don't agree on whether they will work during retirement; 60 percent disagree on the age at which each will retire.[25] There are also indications that blacks and Latinos are less likely to plan for retirement.[26]

But there is also evidence that boomers' personal perceptions of retirement readiness correlate fairly well with more objective economic measures. Two major sample surveys of boomers by AARP (1999, replicated in 2004) and another in 2005 by Merrill Lynch found that approximately 40 percent of boomers felt inadequately prepared for retirement.[27] In the 2004 AARP survey, less than half of respondents described their current financial status as comfortable or well off; nearly 40 percent indicated they were "just making ends meet." Their perceptions were largely validated by an economic risk assessment model by Alicia Munnell et al. estimating that 36 percent of Older Boomers and 43 percent of Younger Boomers were at risk of having inadequate retirement income—even if they worked until age sixty-five.[28] A revised model, adding in health care liabilities, boosted those figures to 50 and 61 percent, respectively.[29]

Health Insurance Anxieties

An increasing number of baby boomers will face retirement and old age with no employer-provided retiree health care benefits; and some of those currently scheduled for such perks are likely to find them greatly reduced. In both the AARP and Merrill Lynch retirement surveys discussed in chapter 1, only half of boomers expected to have health insurance that would meet their needs in retirement. In the 2004 AARP survey, 58 percent of respondents didn't expect employer contributions to their postretirement health insurance; 43 percent didn't expect Medicare to cover most of their medical needs; and 19 percent indicated that they did not expect to have adequate health insurance coverage. The darkest finding was in the Merrill Lynch survey: respondents feared lack of affordable health insurance in retirement (53 percent) more than death itself (17 percent). With good reason: recent estimates suggest that, for the remainder of their life span, a sixty-five-year-old couple will need $240,000 to cover out-of-pocket expenses not covered by Medicare.[30]

Corporations and other private employers have been reducing or eliminating retiree health coverage; the public sector is likely to follow. Even before the onset of the Great Recession, the number of retirees without health insurance rose 25 percent between 2000 and 2005.[31] This is an ominous trend. In surveys by Fidelity Research Institute and the *Wall Street Journal,* about two-thirds of current retirees reported that their monthly expenses were high or higher than expected; increased expenditures for medical and home insurance were the reasons.[32]

A rising medical-technology complex holds out the 1950s advertising slogan of "better living through chemistry" that Older Boomers heard throughout their childhood. Ominously, individual longevity could become a function of what individuals can afford—especially if they do not take care of themselves.

The Focalyst researcher Heather Stern was surprised by the many boomers' self-reported health status. "They're not as healthy as you'd think," she concluded after conducting a massive study of thirty-five thousand Americans over the age of forty-two.[33] Other preliminary studies of aging boomers health confirm Stern's observation. They suggest that aging boomers have health problems equal to or worse than those of their parents at the same age.[34] Many of these chronic conditions are managed with prescription drugs.

Boomers aged fifty-five to sixty-four are already consuming health care in greater amounts than did individuals of the same age in the mid-1990s.[35] And they will undoubtedly watch for and demand evolving, expensive breakthroughs in biotechnology from a Medicare system that already provides far more pharmaceuticals and high-tech treatments than were ever envisioned when the program was founded in 1965. (Medicare recently agreed to pay for bariatric surgery—"stomach banding"—for treatment of type 2 diabetes. Hip and knee replacements have become more routine. And not far in the future is the prospect—and the expense—of growing new organs from an individual's own stem cells.)

But aging boomers' largest unanticipated health care expenses will result from the waning of unpaid family support systems available to previous generations who had more children and stronger kinship bonds.

Fraying Family Safety Nets

> I've never married, have no children and, apart from my mother, do not have a close family. I have a "caretaker" personality, helping elderly neighbors, new parent neighbors, pet owner neighbors (and homeless pets), but there is no one to take care of me. . . . I am downright terrified.
> —Anonymous Web site post quoted by Jane Gross (2008)

Throughout human history, unpaid social support and personal caregiving from family members in old age—often from spouses or daughters—has been the primary source of care for the aged. But the Brookings Institution demographer William Frey points out that fewer older boomers are married and that boomers have had fewer children than previous generations. In 1980, about 66 percent of Americans aged fifty-five to sixty-four lived in married-couple households; by 2005, that figure had dropped to 58 percent. By 2006, 20 percent of U.S. women aged forty to forty-four had never had children, double the percentage in

1978.[36] Up to a third of boomers have had no or only one offspring.[37] Married boomers' families have been weakened by divorce, geographical dispersion, and the isolating effects of younger generations' increasing involvement in Web-based relationships. The rising number of women working full time outside the home also complicates family care networks. Eldercare has joined child care as major problem in balancing work and family. (Adult day care centers and more expensive, individualized home care services are one response.)[38]

Large numbers of childless or divorced boomers are going to face their declining years alone. In terms of sheer numbers, this is something new. Such persons are going to inhabit a late life stage that sociologist Elizabeth Marquardt terms "the New Alone." Children of divorced parents are already experiencing a range of ambivalent emotions and feelings of commitment toward caring for aging, divorced parents. In a recent study on grown children of divorce, Marquardt noted that "much of the expert literature on death and dying implicitly assumes an intact family experience. It assumes that people grow up with their mothers and fathers, who are married to each other when one of them dies. . . . But nearly 40 percent of today's adults have experienced their parents divorce. Increasing numbers of younger adults were born to parents who never married each other at all. . . . The painful contours of the new American way of death will be discovered and defined by my own generation in years to come."[39]

Nor will aging boomers gain family financial support via inheritances. Though the 2004 total value of all U.S. inheritances tripled since the 1970s, the stock market and housing meltdowns have reduced inheritance values, as have lengthening life spans and end-of-life medical costs. Furthermore, unequal concentration of wealth in American society means only a few inheritances will be substantial. Before the 2008 meltdowns, studies by AARP's Public Policy Institute indicated that average inheritances passing to boomers would be about $20,000 to $30,000; the top 5 percent might receive at least $237,000. About 7 percent of all estates contain half of all inherited wealth.[40] (A more optimistic appraisal was offered in a new study by Tiburon Strategic Advisors, which found a median inheritance of $48,000—but only 2 percent receiving above $100,000.)[41]

If aging boomers have fewer of their own children and other family members to support them, how will an increasingly younger nonwhite "Global America" feel about paying medical and retirement bills of a generation of largely white, aging boomers?

OLDER BOOMERS, YOUNGER IMMIGRANTS

"What about immigration?" an AARP board member asked Jacob Hacker after he completed his risk-shift retirement talk to the 2007 AARP Annual Public Policy Meeting. Both Reich's analysis of super-capitalism and Hacker's thesis on risk shift omit mass legal and illegal immigration as potential issues in the future of aging boomers and entitlements. Most analysts do likewise. It's a touchy topic.

Hacker initially seemed a bit surprised and distinctly uneasy—as were several others in the room. "I'm not an expert on immigration," he began. "I'm somewhat conflicted." Finally, Hacker had to admit a basic point avoided in his book: "Social insurance requires membership and boundaries."

That is as far as Hacker and the AARP policy agenda meeting got in approaching a core, but still largely tabooed, contradiction faced by America's policy establishment. On the one hand, they are committed to globalization, transnationalism, and relatively open borders. On the other hand, they wish to maintain relatively generous entitlement programs rooted in the nation-state and the strong national community bond of *E Pluribus Unum*.

Even as immigration policy reform debates erupted anew in 2010, AARP continued its long refusal to comment on the topic. They're not alone. Candid discussion and analyses of immigration and globalization have long been compromised by politically correct pressures to avoid racial stereotypes, positively portray ethnic minorities, "celebrate diversity," and steadfastly support affirmative action policies. The latter, originally designed in the 1960s to remedy past discrimination against blacks, have since expanded to include immigrant minorities under an ambitious new goal: to make American institutions proportionately represent and "look like" the nation's changing demographics.

In the next chapter, I shall discuss in greater detail how immigration and globalization issues are increasingly shaped by competing, class-based worldviews. On the one hand, America's elites favor an internationalist, multicultural outlook congruent with global markets and high immigration levels. This "post-American" viewpoint presumes that the nation-state, national borders, and national identities are passé. On the other hand, middle- and working-class citizens remain wedded to an older worldview rooted in American exceptionalism, economic and cultural nationalism, individual initiative and responsibility, local churches and communities, "family values," and assimilation of limited numbers of legal immigrants.

Immigration in the latter half of the twentieth century was fundamentally changed when Congress passed major immigration reform legislation in 1965. The act eliminated an ethnic quota system that favored European immigrants. In the late 1960s and 1970s immigration to the United States decisively shifted to Third World nations, especially Latin America and the Pacific Rim. Miami and south Florida received increasing numbers of political refugees from Fidel Castro's Cuba, and, by the 1990s, from oppressive Caribbean nations such as Haiti. In the American Southwest, especially in California, the border with Mexico became increasingly porous.

By the mid-1990s, the Brookings Institution demographer William Frey recognized that twenty-first-century America would be shaped by two powerful demographic forces: the aging of the baby boom and the new immigration wave. The dialectic between largely white, aging baby boomers and a younger, far more ethnically diverse "Global America" (to use Frey's phrasing) poses one of the primary challenges to twenty-first-century America.[42]

Frey's findings, supplemented by interviews with U.S. Census officials, led the *New York Times* reporter Sam Roberts to coin the blunt phrase "emerging racial generation gap." In 2007, 80 percent of Americans over age sixty were non-Hispanic whites; they were only 60 percent of those in their twenties and thirties. Half the children under age five were Hispanic, black, or Asian; more than 20 percent of U.S. children were foreign born or had a parent who was. The median age for Hispanics was 27.4; for non-Hispanic whites, 40.5; for the entire U.S. population, 36.6.[43] One year later, Roberts updated this profile with newer Census Bureau findings: racial and ethnic minorities made up 43 percent of Americans under age twenty. In one out of four American counties, black, Hispanic, and Asian children constituted the majority of the under-twenty population.[44] (Parallel economic inequalities along this racial generation gap were suggested by a *USA Today* analysis of Federal Reserve data that found a growing wealth gap between younger and older Americans.[45] And an age-adjusted earnings gap was indicated in a study by the Economic Mobility Project which found that thirty-year-old males today earn less, in inflation-adjusted wages, than did thirty-year-old men during the 1970s.)[46]

Aging boomers and a younger increasingly immigrant America are inextricably linked. Under the terms of the twentieth-century social compact, the old and middle-aged are supposed to fund schools and other public services for young adults and their children; in turn, younger citizens pay for Social Security and Medicare. Changes in boomer family structures combined with mass immigration of younger people from Third World nations into the United States complicate tensions of the traditional "generation gap." As discussed above, compared to their elders, boomers have more attenuated bonds with the future: more of them are single, divorced, or have no children or only one child.

New immigrants and longtime citizen residents may not mix frequently or well. In 2007, the Harvard political scientist Robert Putnam reluctantly published the conclusions from his multicity survey that high levels of immigration-driven ethnic and cultural diversity produced low levels of interpersonal trust and civic engagement—at least in a short to moderately long time frame. Putnam found that "inhabitants of diverse communities tend to withdraw from collective life, to distrust their neighbors, regardless of the color of their skin, to withdraw even from close friends, to expect the worst from their community and its leaders, to volunteer less, to give less to charity and work on community projects less often, to register to vote less . . . to huddle in front of the television. Diversity, at least in the short run, seems to bring out the turtle in all of us."[47]

Two of the cities in Putnam's survey that exemplified his results were Los Angeles and San Francisco, the largest and fourth-largest cities in the nation's increasingly troubled demographic laboratory, California.

AGING BOOMERS IN AMERICA'S TOMORROWLAND

I am one of millions of baby boomers who responded to the seductive message of the Mamas and the Papas' 1960s ballad "California Dreamin.'" I have lived in California for forty years, and it is difficult not to become "California-centric." But it also hard not to notice that the historical arcs of baby boomers—especially the Older Boomers—and California coincide to a great extent. Their affluent postwar past, difficult present, and uncertain future seem to be following parallel trajectories—with very strong implications for the rest of the nation. How aging boomers respond to California's demographic and political changes will determine the outcome of what Peter Schrag has aptly termed "America's Great Experiment."

The Golden State's golden age was the nearly quarter century of post–World War II prosperity, the era of Older Boomers' childhood and adolescence.[48] Buoyed by heavy federal spending on defense and aerospace during World War II and the cold war, the state invested heavily in infrastructure, public schools, and higher education, especially under the early 1960s governor Pat Brown. Millions of Americans were lured west by a California Dream that had always promised a better life for ordinary people, especially the middle class. During this same period, television and rock-and-roll music, increasingly dominated by the Hollywood entertainment complex, molded the youth and cultural consciousness of Older Boomers. California sought to provide universal higher education through construction of a vast, well-funded higher education system, capped by the renowned, multicampus University of California. (The same era, it might be noted, was also the economic heyday for much of America, especially the industrial Midwest—before the slow onset of supercapitalism in the 1970s transformed it into the "Rust Belt.")

Today, both California and aging boomers are more vulnerable in many ways: struggling with near-record levels of unemployment and debt, occupational restructuring, sharp income swings, "deferred maintenance," low or inadequate financial reserves, and uncertain futures. Postwar California's golden era is gone for good. "Pat Brown's California Takes a Beating in Sacramento," lamented the *Los Angeles Times* reporter Cathleen Decker in describing California's battered state budget for 2009.[49]

By 2010, nearly 24.3 percent of the state's population under age sixty-five was without health insurance.[50] A weeklong, free health care clinic held in an Inglewood sports complex drew overflow crowds so large that even veteran California observers used the phrase "Third World" to describe it as a microcosm of statewide inequalities.[51] (Indeed, the clinic organizer, Remote Area Medical, was originally founded to medically minister to Third World nations.) While parts of the nation began to emerge from the Great Recession in mid-2010, California's inland regions still contained twelve of the twenty most economically stressed counties.[52] Not surprisingly, three-quarters of all adults thought the "general direction of things in California" was the "wrong direction," as did 82 percent of voters.[53]

Newsweek's Robert J. Samuelson was one of the first of many observers to call attention to the national implications of California's economic predicament. "There's a collision between high and rising demands for government services and the capacity of the economy to produce the income and tax revenue to pay for those demands. That's true of California, where poor immigrants and their children have increased pressures for more government services. It's also true of the nation, where an aging population raises Social Security and Medicare spending. California is leading the transformation of politics into a form of collective torture: pay more (high taxes) for less (lower services)."[54]

But California's inability to act upon its fiscal problems reflects paralysis resulting from a coalescing, triple age/class/ethnic Sociological San Andreas Fault Line. According to both the University of Southern California policy scholar Dowell Myers and retired *Sacramento Bee* columnist and author Peter Schrag, California's political paralysis and sociological fragmentation result from a disjuncture between the political needs and voting strengths of two different populations: an aging Anglo electorate and a younger, burgeoning, increasingly immigrant general population. This troubling triple divide underpins more oft-mentioned political reasons for California's problems: gerrymandering, powerful public employee unions, "ballot-box budgeting" via dozens of ballot propositions, term limits, a constitutional requirement for a two-thirds majority for passing budgets, and a tax system overly dependent upon the state's wild boom-and-bust swings.[55]

"We are destined to become a state with both a diminishing, rapidly aging white population and a growing, much younger nonwhite population," observes the veteran *Sacramento Bee* columnist Dan Walters. "The declining white population has been politically dominant, accounting for the 70-plus percent of voters, who also tend to be substantially older and more affluent than the population as a whole. And the gap between voters and younger, mostly nonwhite, nonvoting adults has been a continuing headache for the politicians because the two groups' priorities are markedly different."[56]

Non-Hispanic whites' share of California's thirty-six-million population has dropped below 40 percent (below 30 percent of all public school children).[57] Twenty-six percent of Californians were born in another nation—highest amongst all the states; 33 percent of Los Angeles County residents are foreign born, as are 46 percent in the city of Los Angeles.[58] California once was the destination for about 40 percent of all new immigrants; today, approximately 20 percent of all new arrivals to the United States head for the Golden State.[59]

Though California's citizens still perceive a rising immigration tide, Myers contends that the initial immigration wave subsided and leveled off during the 1990s. The second phase of immigrant population growth is being fueled less by immigration and more by high birthrates of those already here. A third phase, just beginning, involves attempts to incorporate immigrants and their children into the political and sociological fabric of the state. This will not be easy.

California has reaped both the benefits and the problems of massive legal and illegal immigration and globalization. Many Asian and Middle Eastern immigrants (and their children) constitute the backbone of small businesses in many cities and older suburbs; they are major players in Silicon Valley and in universities, other research centers, and the state's vast medical and health delivery systems. But though data and measurements are difficult to obtain, illegal immigration has also fueled an expanding underclass complete with shadowy, off-the-books businesses, escalating identity theft and fraud, and crime, especially violent, drug-related street crime in the nation's "gang capital" of Southern California.

Public schools have been on the front lines of demographic change. At least one-fourth of the state's public school children come from homes below the federal poverty line; another one-fourth are English language learners; by some estimates, 40 percent of the Hispanic students in Los Angeles City schools drop out.[60] (A Gates Foundation/

Manhattan Institute study found that 76 percent of California's non-Hispanics whites graduated from high school versus 54 percent of Hispanics and 59 percent of blacks.)[61]

California has tried to equalize public school funding, and it officially ranks in the middle of all fifty states on most measures (per pupil, per capita, etc.). However, wealthier communities have been able to circumvent these efforts by providing substantial private subsidies through 501(c) foundations at many individual schools. In essence, California's public schools are being partially privatized, substantially slowing or reversing equalization efforts. In higher education, by 2010 average state per-student funding at the University of California fell 54 percent from levels in 1991.[62]

The demographic divergence between the general population and an aging electorate began during the 1970s, a decade marked by rising inflation, soaring homeowner tax bills, and rising legal and illegal immigration and capped by the passage of Proposition 13, heralding the "taxpayers' revolt." In addition to freezing property taxes, the measure mandated a two-thirds legislative or voter "supermajority" requirement for future tax increases—further ensuring the continuing dominance of the white electorate. The massive cutbacks in public services and infrastructure forced by Proposition 13 heavily affected schools and other services used by the younger populations of newcomers.[63] In 1994, insult was added to injury when a wide range of voting groups (except Latinos) passed Proposition 187, an initiative denying public services to illegal immigrants (subsequently voided in the courts). That was followed in 1996 by the successful passage of Proposition 209, which outlawed the use of ethnic preferences in public contracting, hiring, and university admissions.

Both Dowell Myers and Peter Schrag mourn the lack of social solidarity, a shared vision of the future that would unite the largely aging and white electorate and younger, struggling minorities. "California's declining sense of community," noted Schrag, "was caused by the withdrawal of a large and growing number of residents into gated privatized residential enclaves and by, on the other hand, the global economic and social relationships in which growing numbers of 'resident expatriates' with dual loyalties and, perhaps dual citizenships, now live."[64]

A more poignant, personal perspective on California's fading future was articulated by Paul Kerkorian, former California Assembly majority leader and currently a member of the Los Angeles City Council. "I grew up when schools were good. The state invested in education under Pat Brown, we built the community college system, the infrastructure, we protected the environment and governed based on what was best for California in the next generation and the next century. That's essentially been wiped from the map now, the idea of working toward a future California my kids will enjoy."[65]

California's ideologically polarized two-party system reflects and reinforces ethnic and civic fragmentation. According to a 2008 Public Policy Institute of California report, the state's Republican Party is 84 percent white, 8 percent Latino, 5 percent Asian, and 1 percent black; for Democrats, the figures are 63 percent white, 20 percent Latino, 5 percent Asian, and 10 percent black. (There is also a moderate difference by gender: women constitute 46 percent of the Republican Party but 57 percent of Democrats.) The Democratic vote is increasingly clustered in urban coastal areas, while the inland areas are more conservative. Ideological polarization between the two parties on a variety of issues has steadily increased, including the question of whether immigrants are a burden or a benefit to society. Fifty-nine percent of Republicans considered immigrants a burden; 32 percent a benefit. Democrats were almost a mirror opposite: 61 percent felt immigrants were a benefit, 30 percent a burden.[66]

Even optimistic boosters of immigration and free-trade globalization, such as the California-based demographer Joel Kotkin, sometimes fret about "the death of the Dream." Kotkin now acknowledges globalization's downside of widening inequalities, polarized politics, and civic malaise. While still harboring hopes for a social contract nourished by a more bipartisan politics, Kotkin fears that the increasing economic and ethnic divisions in the state may be both deep and permanent.[67] Echoing Schrag and Myers, Kotkin warns that "a generational conflict is brewing, pitting the interests and predilections of well-heeled boomers against a growing, predominately Latino working class. . . . The only way out of this looming crisis lies with the boomer gentry doing something totally out of character: getting past their self-interest and self-love for the good of the next generation. . . . If not, their Eden will end up as a green version of a gated community."[68]

The well-known California historian Kevin Starr concurs: "Why is it 50 or 60 years ago, we had the capacity to lay down the physical, psychological, cultural, public infrastructure of a global mega-state and today we are on the verge of being Honduras?"[69] And the United States is becoming more like California.

CALIFORNIA'S DEMOGRAPHIC AND POLITICAL DIVIDES GO NATIONAL

If California's demographic changes, economic crises, and polarized political landscape seem increasingly familiar to national political analysts, they should. The twin demographic revolutions of aging boomers and immigration-driven ethnic change that have transformed California are also changing the nation's sociological landscape. By the summer of 2010, the U.S. Census Bureau was reporting that nearly half of all births in the United States were to nonwhite minorities.[70]

The Brookings demographer William Frey has discerned three distinct emerging demographic subregions: (1) Multicultural America, which includes the immigrant magnet areas of California, New York, Texas, and Illinois; (2) the predominantly white, fast-growing Sunbelt, a broadly L-shaped pattern of states that includes much of the Rocky Mountains, the Southwest, and the Southeast; and (3) the Heartland of Great Plains and upper Midwest and border states, which have comparatively low rates of international or domestic in-migration and are largely white and aging more rapidly than the other regions. Frey found that "presenior" baby boomers were migrating to bustling here-tofore youthful Sunbelt areas such as Dallas, Atlanta, Austin, and Las Vegas. Yet "aging in place" will also continue. By 2020, Georgia's senior population will grow by 40 percent, and some states in the Heartland will age even more rapidly because of out-migration of younger citizens and very low in-migration.[71] (Though there was some dispersion of immigrant minorities early in the new century, Frey recently found that there was a renewed trend back to the traditional "gateway cities" of Los Angeles, New York, and Miami.)[72]

California's class-based, progressive-versus-populist responses to demographic changes and economic polarization also look increasingly familiar in national politics. (The history of this national division—and its effect on aging boomer political solidarity—will be discussed further in chapter 3.)

California's corporate and political elites, as well as many of its upper-middle-class professionals, have promoted progressive, big-government proposals to reform tax and budget restrictions and to rebuild public infrastructure, especially schools, health care, roads, and the criminal justice system. In 2000, this coalition sponsored a successful state ballot initiative that relaxed the two-thirds majority requirement for passing local school bond issues.[73] The state's latest budget crisis has opened the door once again to liberal reform groups such as California Forward and Repair California, which have tried to sponsor ballot propositions that would convene a constitutional convention.[74]

This coalition of elites and professionals implicitly or explicitly endorses what Dowell Myers terms a "new social contract" that emphasizes the mutual interests of aging whites and younger immigrants. The aging white electorate will allegedly benefit from creating an educated, young, minority middle-class workforce and taxpayer base that, ultimately, can sustain prosperity and eventually purchase aging boomers' real estate. Higher immigrant birthrates will stabilize population aging and possible decline through lower birthrates for citizens.[75]

But Peter Schrag sensed a deep and powerful source of resistance. "The correspondence between rising immigration and declining services certainly reinforces the research and simple logic which indicate that when the beneficiaries are the voters or their children, voters are likely to be more enthusiastic about services than when the beneficiaries are someone else's children, especially if the someone else is an illegal immigrant."[76] Mass legal and illegal immigration, Schrag predicted, would reenergize antitax populism. And indeed it has—in California and throughout the nation.

In 2003, when the increasingly unpopular California governor Gray Davis proposed granting drivers' licenses to illegal aliens, he triggered a successful recall movement driven by heavily white, middle-aged, middle-class populists who were also instrumental in electing his "no-new-taxes" replacement, Republican Arnold Schwarzenegger. (And in 2009, when Schwarzenegger reneged on his no-new-taxes pledge by endorsing ballot proposals to raise taxes, California's populist antitax forces rallied to defeat them.)[77]

California's long-simmering populist anger over the impact of illegal immigration in California surged nationwide in 2007. Fueled by talk radio and the Internet, this grassroots protest movement swamped congressional telephone systems and killed a major immigration reform bill being rushed through the U.S. Senate by a bipartisan coalition backed by the Bush White House. This new populism has revealed a new "generation gap" over immigration: white boomers and older Americans are the age groups most opposed to lax immigration enforcement; young people are far less concerned.[78]

By July 2010, the spread to the national level of California's demographic and political trends had become the topic of Ronald Brownstein's *National Journal* article, "The Gray and the Brown: A Generational Mismatch." Echoing Frey's analyses, Brownstein portrayed a potential clash of national priorities between a graying population that is nearly 80 percent white and a population under age eighteen that is 56 percent minority. The older population will be wary of public spending on anything other than old age entitlements, while younger Americans will favor increased spending for schools, health, social welfare programs, and infrastructure.[79]

The real estate meltdown, the stock market crash, the Great Recession, rising resentment about high public-sector pay and pensions, and the narrow passage of national health care reform also completed the nationalization of California populism via the "Tea Party" movement. Like California's antitax, antigovernment, anti–illegal immigration, anti–race quota populism, the Tea Party has been rooted in its middle-aged and older white working and middle classes (They are a major audience demographic of talk radio, a major purveyor of "class consciousness" for the new populism. Many new populists are at home with the Web, the Internet, and cell phone technologies that enhance rapid communication and organization.)[80]

In California and ultimately the rest of the nation, however, relentless demographic change will favor the "new social contract" progressivism promoted by white boomer elites and will diminish middle-class white, boomer-driven populism.[81] California's electorate is becoming younger and more heavily minority, mirroring the general population. This is occurring through the exodus of nearly half a million whites from 2000 to 2008 along with the rise in naturalized citizens who are mostly Latino and Asian—almost three hundred thousand in 2008.[82] Polling data suggest that they are likely to favor greater investment in schools and the rest of public infrastructure even if it means higher taxes.[83] Registration is plummeting for California's largely white and aging Republican Party with a statewide record low of 31 percent in 2009. Not a single congressional, state, or assembly district had a majority Republican registration.[84]

These demographic divides will exacerbate an already-evident public policy tug-of-war within California state and local government between greater education and social services spending for younger families with children versus pension, health care, and retiree benefits for older Californians.

On both the state and national levels, this spreading age/class/ethnicity Sociological San Andreas Fault Line rumbles ominously for aging boomers. Whether aging boomers will politically mobilize to defend entitlements and other public spending on their behalf is the subject of the next chapter.

CHAPTER THREE

Boomers' Senior Power Potential

From Social Protest to Self-Preservation

Generational tension, and maybe generational war, is an
inevitable part of the Age of Obama.
> —*Newsweek* (January 17, 2009)

The modern history of old age politics is far more complex,
and the future will not be as scary as some predict.
> —James Schulz and Robert Binstock (2006)

In February 2007, a key Republican political tactician, whom I
shall call "the Strategist," told me he had given little or no thought
to aging baby boomers as a political force. Age-based voting was
not an especially important factor on Republicans' political radar
screen—nor were Democratic strategists considering aging boomers'
political potential.

"We look at the data," the Strategist told me. "By numbers, boomers
are the 'pig in the python.' But that's about it. They've not been through
a cohesive, transformational threat. On the political side, they're a difficult group to categorize." He paused and then added, "The one unifying thing about boomers is their sense of entitlement," especially with
regard to Social Security. The Republican voter strategy, he informed
me, was values driven. "We look at religion, education, family. Married
or not married."

Winter daylight streaming through high windows in the Strategist's huge, high-ceilinged executive office building suite dimmed dramatically. Outside, a heavy shower of sleet and snow started to shut down Washington, D.C., and much of the East Coast. Federal employees and many other political appointees left work early. The Strategist and his aides remained at their posts. As his other afternoon appointments canceled, my original forty-five-minute interview drifted into a two-hour conversation.

We discussed the administration's failed Social Security reform initiative. The Strategist admitted some polling evidence of different generational responses to the initiative—reflecting a pattern typically found among age groups. Those aged sixty and above wanted no change. Those aged forty-five to fifty-two were nervous. Younger voters "mouthed the arguments [in favor of personalized Social Security accounts] but didn't care."

The Strategist echoed a growing Washington lament on entitlement reform in an era of polarization. "Politics trumps long-term planning." Rather prophetically, he added that "only a major crisis would prompt serious change."

When I asked him about AARP, the Strategist's eyes narrowed. He became animated. "They are evil!" he snorted. He went on to say that the Bush White House felt double-crossed by the giant lobbying organization. AARP had worked cooperatively with the White House in enacting the 2003 Medicare Modernization Act that added prescription drug coverage to Medicare. But then, after some positive overtures on similar cooperation on Social Security reform, AARP instead worked hard to torpedo Bush's effort to institute private Social Security accounts.

The Strategist grumbled that behind closed doors AARP officials admitted serious, long-term fiscal problems with Social Security. Publicly, however, they claimed that only minor tinkering with the program was needed. The Strategist sneered at AARP's CEO Bill Novelli for "hiding behind their president [Marie Smith], a leftist, radical woman."

Like several other Republicans to whom I spoke, he complained that the left-wing, pro–big government AARP "leverages their marketing for political purposes."

When I mentioned the potential convergence of interests between aging boomers and AARP, the Strategist considered this as if for the first time. He became intrigued and we talked about a boomer-AARP alliance for several minutes. "AARP," he mused, "could create generational politics."[1] Indeed, they already had.

Boomers responded strongly in support of AARP's campaign against George W. Bush's efforts to introduce "personalized" accounts into the Social Security system.[2] The Democratic Party consultants Greenberg Quinlin Rosner, in a 2005 voter attitude survey, also found the most negative responses to Bush's proposals by voters in their fifties—older baby boomers.[3]

Well before the 2008 stock market crash and Great Recession there were rumblings of anxiety and discontent among baby boomers. A boomer profile by McKinsey and Company found that many "are anxious, frustrated, more concerned about their future than were members of the previous generation."[4] Career consultant Andrew Johnson also sensed an underlying anxiety about Social Security among his upscale clients in real estate and banking. Boomers, Johnson stated, saw Social Security as the last remaining certainty in an increasingly insecure workplace and world. "Boomers seem to think that it's nice to know that there's something you can depend on."[5]

Boomers' parents and grandparents felt the same way—and became feared as a formidable "senior vote," a potentially unified force allegedly ready to terminate the career of any politician who touched the "third rail" of Social Security or Medicare cutbacks. But was this fear justified?

Some social scientists argue that age is not a significant factor in political behavior and that senior power is something of a myth. And baby boomers' senior power potential has yet to show itself in that generation's earlier voting patterns.

BOOMERS AND AGE-BASED POLITICS

Before discussing the relationship between age and politics, it is necessary to note the extensive overlap of age, race, and the baby boom—implicit throughout this book. In discussing the white eligible-voter population, the Brookings Institution demographer William Frey emphasized the correlation of "white" with "age"—largely due to the dominance of the boomers: "An attribute of the white eligible-voter population that distinguishes it from the other eligible-voter populations is its age. More dominated by baby boomers than the other groups, over half are over age forty-five and nearly a fifth are over age sixty-five. Compared with the total eligible-voter population, whites are more educated, have higher incomes and are more likely to be married and are almost universally native-born. But it is their age more than any other attribute that drives their demographic profile."[6]

As seen in chapter 1, about 24 percent of Older Boomers are black, Hispanic, and Asian, as are 27 percent of Younger Boomers. However, minority boomers are rarely subcategorized in age-based data; indeed, until recently, the boomer age demographic (roughly ages forty-five to sixty-four) was imprecisely referenced, if at all. Therefore, throughout this book, unless otherwise noted, discussions of "boomer politics" and "age politics" will refer, somewhat by default, largely to the political behavior and attitudes of non-Hispanic whites.

As a whole, boomers have not yet voted as a distinctive generational "bloc," though Duane F. Alwin detected broad, distinctive generational response patterns to survey items included in the University of Michigan National Election Studies during the 1980s and 1990s. Those findings confirmed boomers' increasingly conservative, antigovernment attitudes (discussed in the previous chapter).[7] John B. Williamson concurred and, consequently, saw little possibility of any aging boomer activism: "It is unlikely that there will be a sharp increase in political activism among the baby boomers as they move into old age," in part because the increasing heterogeneity and inequality among boomers will make organizational efforts more difficult. Nonetheless, Williamson held out the possibility of aging boomer activism in three potent policy arenas: Social Security, Medicare, and school taxation.[8]

Nor have boomers had a distinctive presence in presidential election voting. The boomer age group has generally mirrored the wider electorate—never decisively favoring any candidate. A majority of boomers voted for Ronald Reagan but then slightly tilted leftwards toward Bill Clinton. They gave George W. Bush small majorities in the 2000 and 2004 presidential elections. In 2008, boomers as a whole were evenly split between presidential candidates Barack Obama and John McCain by 50 percent to 49 percent—though white boomers gave McCain a 56 percent-42 percent margin.

Aging boomers have been increasingly attentive to Social Security and Medicare. The 2004 AARP "Boomers at Midlife" survey found that 71 percent of respondents reported at least a "somewhat favorable" view of Social Security (up 15 percent from a similar 2002 survey); 54 percent were very or somewhat confident that Social Security would be available when they retired (up 19 percent); and 47 percent were at least somewhat confident that they would receive Medicare (up 8 percent).[9] Nearly 90 percent of boomer respondents in a 2005 Merrill Lynch survey of boomers agreed that their generation was fully entitled to Medicare and Social Security; 80 percent felt the same about prescription drug coverage.[10] And, as already mentioned, many boomers opposed George W. Bush's 2005 proposed changes to Social Security.

By 2009, an important change was occurring. Higher than expected numbers of baby boomers turning age sixty-two were filing for early Social Security benefits. This marked an ongoing generational transition from anticipating entitlements to "owning" them—and, perhaps, mobilizing politically to protect them.

But has *any* previous cohort of those over age sixty-five ever truly constituted a unified or voting bloc or political force? Or is senior power something of a myth?

SENIOR POWER: MYTH OR SLEEPING GIANT?

The assumption of older voters' actual or potential political power is premised upon their higher political participation rates—often attributed to increased leisure time in retirement, long-term residence, and increased attention to news media. That older voters' dependence upon and interest in preserving Social Security and Medicare policies might explain their higher voting rates as a "program constituency" was a thesis advanced by Andrea Louise Campbell in *How Policies Make Citizens*.[11] She argued that the advent and the expansion of first Social Security and then Medicare served to mobilize older citizens into a bloc of "Uber-citizens . . . an otherwise disparate group of people were given a new political identity as program recipients that provided a basis for their mobilization by political parties, interest groups and policy entrepreneurs."[12] Social Security benefits provided resources (income and free time) as well as the motivation to politically participate. Government policy became connected to seniors' financial well-being.

Though Campbell discerned seniors' rising awareness and participation, she did not demonstrate that they voted as a cohesive bloc—or that their voting patterns were significantly different from other groups. However, Campbell got closer to the source of "senior power" imagery by factoring into her model the rise of senior citizens' interest groups as well as growth of a government-based "aging policy bureaucracy." These organizations and the major political parties, rather than a unified senior voting bloc, strongly shaped past congressional perception and action on aging policies.

Robert Binstock has been the foremost critic of what he views as a mythical "senior power model" that presumes the primacy of age-based self interest in voting behavior that, in turn, produces a unified senior voting bloc. Binstock argues that empirical analyses of voting behavior find that voters' choices are more often determined by factors other than age—such as socioeconomic status, gender, race, ethnicity, religion, and health status. Divisions among senior voters often mirror those among other age groups. Therefore, Binstock concludes, "The senior power model has little validity with respect to the political attitudes and voting behavior of older Americans, and only limited validity with respect to the power of U.S. old-age organizations."[13] In addition, he argues, the model exaggerates the influence and effectiveness of senior citizen interest groups such as AARP.

In their 2006 book *Aging Nation,* Binstock and coauthor James Schulz still maintained that there had been little evidence of age-based voting blocs. They also maintained that there was no systematic evidence that older voters had ever responded as a distinctive voting group to old-age policy issues (Medicare and Social Security).[14] However, they admitted that senior power had remained a sleeping giant because of politicians' fear of awakening it—especially through active discussions of Social Security and Medicare reforms: "Candidates are on the ballot, but issues affecting Social Security, Medicare and other national old-age policies are not."[15]

Obviously, things have changed.

In 2009, threats to Medicare became a hot-button political issue when a five-hundred-billion-dollar reduction in its rate of growth was incorporated in the Patient Protection and Affordable Care Act that narrowly passed the Congress in 2010. Some Republicans began to champion Medicare by invoking a fear of "death panels" and evoking imagery of rationed health care for the elderly. As will be discussed in greater detail in chapter 6, voters over age fifty were (and remain) the most vocally opposed to Democrats' health care reform proposals and were active in the spontaneous town hall protests in August 2009. These outbursts of collective protest behavior spurred the rise of the loosely organized "Tea Party movement," in which older baby boomer whites have been heavily involved.

Before briefly discussing the Tea Party movement at the end of the chapter, it is necessary to examine a broader, key question in this chapter and in this book: whether there is yet a sufficient fusion of ideological consensus and collective economic convergence to galvanize a "critical mass" of Older Boomers into becoming a visible voting bloc or a more organized and active political movement. (The important potential leadership role of AARP in these policy debates will be discussed in chapters 5 and 6.)

CONSENSUS AND CONVERGENCE?

Two key social psychological processes underpin mobilization and movement building. First, preexisting or socially constructed *consensus* on basic values and norms facilitates communication and interaction. Second, mobilization and organization are enhanced when there is *convergence* of similar interests and background characteristics—such as shared economic interests or shared sociological characteristics (gender, ethnicity, age, religion, region, etc.).[16]

In this chapter I shall examine evidence for and against cultural and ideological consensus among boomers. The prospects for economic convergence through shared risk in retirement and health care planning (or lack thereof) were touched upon in the previous chapter. The case for even greater convergence of economic interest and vulnerability in the wake of the 2008 stock market crash and the long Great Recession will be discussed in chapter 4. (Suffice it to say here that these events intensified aging boomers' collective economic anxieties.)

In terms of cultural or ideological consensus, however, boomers' fierce "do-it-yourself" individualism and an ideological divide rooted in class, occupation, education, and culture, may be potent factors blocking emergence of an age-based voting bloc or a more active, organized political movement based upon shared economic interests or anxieties.

In chapter 1 it was made clear that boomers, especially Older Boomers, accept their generational label and a loose age-based identity. They have much in common culturally, especially nostalgia for the music and popular culture of their youth. They are relatively ethnically homogeneous. They share a broad cultural base rooted in a childhood and adolescent history defined by prosperity, the cold war, relative ethnic homogeneity (due to low immigration levels), and a culture largely programmed by three national television networks and the rise of a formidable music radio and record industry. Older Boomers, especially, share passage through the political crucibles of the JFK assassination, the Vietnam War, and the Watergate scandal. They have participated in massive institutional change at work and at home.

The impact of the "culture wars" stemming from the Vietnam War and other 1960s changes has been much debated in the media and social sciences. Some analysts, notably Alan Wolfe in *One Nation after All,* have argued that the culture wars have been overemphasized in the mass media. Wolfe argued that there is a broad moral and value consensus across most groups on a wide range of issues in American society.[17]

The 2008 elections strongly suggest that any broad, national moral and value consensus has absorbed the reformist goals and spirit of the 1960s movements. Peter Beinart vividly illustrated this accommodation by comparing the violent street protests at the 1968 Democratic Convention to the 2008 peaceful celebration of President Barack Obama's election—and ideological change—in that same Chicago Grant Park setting: "Ideologically, the crowds who assembled to hear Obama on election night were linear descendants of those egg throwers four decades before. They too believe in racial equality, gay rights, feminism, civil liberties and people's right to follow their own star. . . . Feminism is so mainstream that even Sarah Palin embraces the term; Chicago mayor Richard Daley, son of the man who told police to bash heads, marches in gay-rights parades. . . . Younger Americans—who voted overwhelmingly for Obama—largely embrace the legacy of the '60s, and yet they constitute one of the most obedient, least rebellious generations in memory."[18]

Whatever the impact of the 1960s and its culture wars, once youthful boomers are today crossing a number of "senior citizen" markers that signal increasing risk of mortality: early warning signals of chronic disease or its actual onset; rising problems with employer-based health insurance costs; the temptation of "senior citizen" discounts; and increasing awareness of personal mortality and awakening desires to leave enduring legacies. These passages were increasing age consciousness even before the economic shocks of 2008 and beyond.

Yet thus far aging boomers have responded as individuals. Their youthful calls for egalitarian, collective change seem a distant echo. Today, some issues engage aging boomers; others do not.

A POLITICS OF TAILORED ENGAGEMENT

What is remarkable is that multiple shocks of the stock market crash, the real estate collapse, mass layoffs, and other aspects of what has come to be known as the Great Recession have not stimulated any sort of mass, left-wing protests advocating major changes in the system that led to these crises. The Obama White House and Democratic Congress enacted major progressive reforms of the health care and financial systems. But there are no broadly based 1960s-style egalitarian movements to redistribute wealth and power or to reverse the Great Risk Shift in retirement and health care costs to individuals.

Nor has age discrimination against graying boomers produced a "new civil rights movement"—as some had hoped. The deep and long recession unquestionably has made boomers far more aware of their vulnerability to age discrimination: in 2008, age discrimination complaints to the Equal Employment Opportunity Commission soared—up 29 percent over the previous year.[19] Yet the mass filing of *individual* age discrimination complaints hardly constitutes *collective* outrage or protest.

Indeed, on June 18, 2009, a potentially galvanizing Supreme Court decision made it more difficult for plaintiffs to prove age discrimination. In *Gross v. FBL Financial Services,* the court reversed an earlier appellate court age discrimination standard that if a worker could demonstrate that age was one of many factors, then the employer was required to provide a reason unrelated to age. Justice Clarence Thomas's 5–4 majority opinion now requires that the plaintiff must definitively prove that age was *the* primary factor in workplace discrimination.

With the exception of an initial, long front-page report on the *Gross* decision by the *Los Angeles Times*'s David Savage, there was little substantial acknowledgement elsewhere.[20] Nor was there an immediate call to arms on the AARP Web page—which simply provided a link to Savage's article. Instead, it was nearly a month before the *New York Times* lead editorial coupled notice and criticism of the ruling with a call for congressional repeal.[21] More than a year later, despite quiet efforts in Congress to draft legislation mitigating the *Gross* decision (heavily supported by AARP), the case still generates little interest.

Aging boomers' continuing ideological emphases upon individual actions and responsibility short-circuit the shared group communication and political consciousness-raising that promote a sense that "something needs to be done," necessary ingredients for collective action and systematic reform. Even during the pessimism and hardships of the Great Recession, a 2010 Allstate-National Journal heartland monitor poll found that Americans were responding with a "back to basics" emphasis on individual responsibility, financial management, and frugality; they were less confident in American institutions and leadership.[22]

Thus age discrimination and the Great Recession's massive job losses have been met with personal alienation, blame, and shame. "For weeks after he was laid off, Clinton Cole would rise at the usual time, shower, shave, and don one of his Jos. A Bank suits and head out the door of his Vienna home—to a job that no longer existed. He was careful to stay away until 5 p.m., whiling away the hours at the library or on a park bench. . . . Cole was too ashamed to tell anyone except his wife and family what had happened. . . . He felt as if he had done something wrong, even though he knew he hadn't."[23] In another *Washington Post* report on the recession's impact upon wealthy New York suburbs, three dozen mostly middle-aged residents interviewed for the story refused to permit publication of their names or identifying details.[24] (A subsequent survey of the long-term unemployed by the Rutgers University Center for Workforce Development confirmed escalating levels of individual stress, depression, self-blame, and social withdrawal.)[25]

The complete lack of collective response to layoffs, high unemployment levels, and age discrimination stands in sharp contrast to the uproar among Americans over age fifty generated by health care reform. One example: on the AARP Web page, a defense of Democratic health care reform proposals by AARP's president was met with a storm of nearly one thousand mostly angry responses; an article on that same Web site concerning an age discrimination lawsuit against AT&T drew only three reader comments.[26] (Indeed, as will be seen in chapter 6, AARP officials were dismayed to discover that opposition was strongest among their own constituency.)

This selective, issue-oriented, highly individualized boomer politics was predicted by a 2004 AARP study entitled *A Changing Political Landscape*. Though completed well before the current economic traumas, the authors concluded that boomers' common cultural heritage would not be sufficient to generate a voting bloc or a rerun of 1960s mass-movement protests. Instead, aging boomer politics would be issue oriented, reflecting a more limited political style of "tailored engagement," operating outside the traditional two-party system via Web-based communities and "checkbook activism."[27] Boomers' "strong sense of entitlement and self-directed motivations will help to create a more decentralized, broader, community-based path for activism."[28]

Any tendencies toward unified Boomer consensus in values and politics is also being fragmented by broader sociological variables: (1) socioeconomic status, (2) ethnicity, (3) educational levels, (4) age subgroups—Older and Younger Boomers have somewhat different life experiences, (5) family status—married versus unmarried, children versus no children; (6) regional differences, (7) religious differences, and (7) lingering cultural/political divisions from the 1960s.

But the 2008 elections strongly suggest that cultural and political differences today are less about well-worn debates over issues from the

1960s than about a widening class-based cultural divide. Past arguments about abortion and affirmative action linger, but, increasingly, debates are grounded in a clash of class-based worldviews. The key debate here is the increasing influence of global supercapitalism versus the waning influence and identity of local communities and the nation-state.

A CLASS-BASED POLITICAL/CULTURAL DIVIDE

The relationship between income, assets, and retirement outlook was evident in the AARP and Merrill Lynch studies discussed in chapter 1. Indeed, a broader and deeper class, political, and cultural divide is increasingly structuring American politics in general and boomers' politics in particular. Along with their commitment to individualism, this class/political/cultural divide is the factor most likely to thwart the consensus and convergence necessary to produce a boomer voting bloc or political movement.

Just as Older Boomers moved into their most productive years during the 1980s and 1990s, technology, globalization, and immigration transformed the American middle class into two polarized subclasses.[29] Generally speaking, there has been a growing, politically liberal, highly educated, globally oriented, prosperous upper middle class rooted in the professional and managerial occupations, often residents of major urban areas on the East or West Coast—or in university enclaves.[30] Their multicultural and international worldview and policy predilections for top-down "management" of societal problems through social engineering are typically opposed by those who are to be managed: a declining lower middle and working class that is primarily white, without college degrees, culturally conservative, nationalistic, locally oriented, and antielitist and that tends to be made up of (traditional) "values voters." Their presence is especially strong in the nation's interior: the midwestern heartland, the South and Southwest, and the mountain states. (Most of the "battleground states" in the 2008 elections were in these regions.)

All Americans have been affected by this major change in social stratification, but boomers were at the epicenter of this sociological earthquake. "Over the past 20 years," observed Harvard political scientist Robert Putnam, "college-educated white people with above average income have become happier, more optimistic and more trusting, even as their fellow citizens in the lower quarter of the social economic pyramid have grown less happy, less optimistic and less trusting."[31]

Several scholars have charted the growth and characteristics of a new globally oriented upper middle class. Christopher Lasch, in his 1995 classic *The Revolt of the Elites*, observed that members of "the upper middle class, the heart of the new professional and managerial elites," have a distinctive outlook and lifestyle that sets them apart from the rest of the nation. Their fortunes and loyalties are tied to international enterprises, and they have "more in common with their counterparts in Brussels or Hong Kong than with the masses of Americans not yet plugged into the network of global communications."[32]

Likewise, Robert Kaplan in *An Empire Wilderness* found that "as the income gap widens, the American middle class continues to split into an increasingly rarified upper middle class and an increasingly downtrodden lower middle class as the middle slowly fades into one or the other."[33] The new upper middle class has increasingly segregated itself into semi-self-contained suburban "pods" that "are creating an international civilization influenced by the impersonal, bottom-line values of the corporations for which these people work."[34] Via computers and satellites, the professional classes are far more involved with national and international peers; they may have little or no familiarity with—and little interest in—local groups or local government. National interests and loyalties are submerged in global concerns. "Rather than citizens, the inhabitants of these prosperous pods are, in truth, resident expatriates, even if they were born in America, with their foreign cuisines, eclectic tastes, exposure to foreign languages, and friends throughout the world."[35]

These professional and managerial classes quite naturally have a deep and abiding faith in their ability to rationally manage human affairs. Indeed, Older Boomers came of age during the ascent of "the best and the brightest" ethos—a faith in meritocracy and managerial hubris enshrined in 1960s Kennedy administration.[36] Forty years later, the writer Joan Didion observed that her upper-middle-class friends "shared a habit of mind usually credited to the very successful. They believed absolutely in their own management skills." All problems could be solved by the right expert with the proper information.[37]

Boomers Bill Clinton and Bill Gates are exemplars of this managerial, globally oriented class. Their vast philanthropic efforts are international. The *New York Times* columnist Tom Friedman epitomizes such views in his columns and in his books, notably *The World Is Flat*. America's cultural, political, and commercial elites champion—or, at least, quietly accept—multiculturalism, high immigration levels, and affirmative action.[38]

In its most aggressive forms, this upper-middle-class worldview hardens into a more dogmatic "political correctness," an aggressive form of censorship and labeling as "racist" or "reactionary" those with dissident views. Targets often have been middle-aged and older white middle- and working-class voters. (See chapter 4.) For more than twenty years, this elites-masses clash has appeared most vividly in polling data and in heated rhetoric over multicultural and social engineering issues such as affirmative action and immigration reform.[39]

The American working and middle classes (including many immigrant groups) tend to maintain an older worldview centered on beliefs in American exceptionalism; economic and cultural nationalism; individual initiative and responsibility rooted in local churches, schools, and communities; and "family values." They believe in "free enterprise" and the hope of upward mobility. By and large, the white middle-aged and older middle classes are part of a nationalist "Old America" that mistrusts, and in some cases has been economically wounded by, the elites' prescriptions for an internationalist "New America." They reject the elites' multiculturalism and believe that immigrants should assimilate to "American" values.

· The *Wall Street Journal* columnist and former Ronald Reagan speechwriter Peggy Noonan has been attuned to the values and fears of many middle- and working-class Americans. "So many Americans right now fear that they are losing their country, that the old America is slipping away and being replaced by something worse, something formless and hollowed out. They can see we are giving up our sovereignty, that our leaders will not control our borders and that we don't teach the young the old-fashioned love of America, that the government has taken to itself such power, and made things so complex, and at the end of the day when they count up sales tax, property tax, state tax they are paying a lot of money to lose the place they loved."[40]

This widening class/political/cultural divide has been evident in the voting and political behavior of boomers and other Americans. They have been part of a central political paradox noted by Democratic strategists Stanley Greenberg and James Carville:[41] though college-educated, upper-income voters remain Republican in presidential elections, Democratic candidates have been gaining a greater percentage of them; meanwhile, the white working classes, once the backbone of the Democratic Party, have trended toward Republican, antitax, traditionalist, "strong defense" candidates—at the apparent expense of their own economic interests.[42] Again, this divide appears to have begun within—and remained deepest in—the baby boom generation.

Alan Abramowitz and Ruy Teixeira studied the voting divide between the rising upper middle class and the declining white working class largely through the variable of college/noncollege. Beginning in 1984, disaffected non-college-educated whites became "Reagan Democrats," in presidential campaigns. By 2004 "among non-college-educated whites with $30,000-$50,000 in household income Bush beat Kerry by 24 points (62–38). . . . And among non-college-educated whites with $50-$75,000 in household income, Bush beat Kerry by a shocking

41 points (70–29)." The defection of the white working class was especially steep in the South.[43]

In 2004, John Kerry won college-educated white voters at the $50,000 to $75,000 household income level by 5 percent. Above the $100,000 income threshold, Bush won college graduates by 60 to 39 percent; but he won those with advanced degrees by only 51 to 48 percent.[44] (Slightly different findings resulted when Brady et al. used occupational groupings rather than education to demarcate the white working class. From 1972 to 1992, the white working-class vote mirrored the general electorate. After 1996, white working-class men did indeed shift to Republicans; white working-class women did not.)[45]

Along with race and age, this trend strongly structured baby boomer voting in the 2008 presidential election and afterwards in attitudes toward President Obama and in the 2010 national congressional races.[46] The youngest and oldest voters also voted distinctively. Younger voters voted 2–1 for Democrat Barack Obama. Voters over sixty-five were the only age group who favored McCain.

THE OBAMA CANDIDACY SPLITS THE BOOMERS

Upscale, well-educated whites—many of them boomers—were essential builders of the Obama political coalition. Indeed, before the primary voting began, many boomers in the major news media and political establishments helped pave the path for the Obama bandwagon. The white working and middle classes tended to prefer Hillary Clinton or John McCain.

"Goodbye to All That" was Andrew Sullivan's parting shot at polarized boomer politics in his *Atlantic* cover story on December 7, 2007. The influential writer and blogger proclaimed that "Obama is the only candidate who can take America—finally—past the debilitating, self-perpetuating family quarrel of the Baby Boom generation." Obama's very face, waxed Sullivan, would lead to the most effective "re-branding" of America to the rest of the world since Reagan. As president, Obama's multiethnic, multinational heritage would ipso facto give the lie to international terrorism's portrait of a racist America "in a way that no words can." In symbol and style, an Obama presidency had the potential to transcend religious, racial, and generational divides. "We may in fact have finally found that bridge to the 21st century that Bill Clinton told us about," gushed Sullivan. "His name is Obama."[47]

The baby boomer daughter and granddaughter of two former iconic presidents boarded the Obama bandwagon. "We need a change in the leadership of this country—just as we did in 1960," wrote Caroline Kennedy in a *New York Times* op-ed. "All my life, people have told me that my father changed their lives . . . and the generation he inspired has passed that spirit on to his children. . . . As parents, we have a responsibility to help our children to believe in themselves and in their power to shape their future. Senator Obama is inspiring my children, my parents' grandchildren, with that sense of possibility."[48] (Her uncle, Senator Ted Kennedy, simultaneously endorsed Obama.) One week later Susan Eisenhower published her endorsement in a *Washington Post* op-ed.[49]

The Generation X political journalist Matt Bai applauded this welcome generational leadership change in the *New York Times Magazine*. "For those of us Obama's age and younger, the formative events of the 1960s, the enmities and shared experiences that defined the next 40 years of American politics are as much a part of history as the Treaty of Versailles; we weren't shaped by this constant sense of political Armageddon. . . . But from here out . . . the balance will shift until ultimately the 'Top Gun' generation has pushed aside the boomer establishment."[50]

Obama's main antagonist, baby boomer Hillary Clinton, was dismayed to find herself portrayed as a symbol of the past. "The Boomers Had Their Day, Make Way for the Millennials," trumpeted a *Washington Post* op-ed by Morley Winograd and Michael D. Hais in February 2008. Obama was identifying Clinton with the older, idealistic "'Moses generation'" that led the children of Israel out of slavery, while aligning himself with the more practical "'Joshua Generation'" that actually built the Kingdom of Israel. This was an "election battle that's being fought along the dividing line between these two generational archetypes."[51]

"Clinton is what our country has been," a Harvard law student told *New York Times* columnist Roger Cohen. "She's not where we're going, which is more diverse, more global, with fewer expectations about what it means to be black or white."[52]

But many aging boomers were not pleased to have their generation's politics and politicians consigned to the past. Former President Bill Clinton bristled at such suggestions by PBS interviewer Charlie Rose.

> CHARLIE ROSE: And when people say we need to go beyond looking back at the '60s or even the '90s, then you say, "I think a lot of good things happened in the '60s, and I think a lot of good things happened in the '70s, in the 80s and the '90s."
>
> BILL CLINTON: If that's relevant. Look at this decade. Look at this record. She [Hillary Clinton] has been a completely modern senator. She has sponsored—she just passed a bill, as a candidate for president, with Lindsay Graham who led my—who was one of the impeachment managers, to extend the family and medical leave law to the families of veterans who were suffering physical and emotional trauma in Iraq or Afghanistan. I mean that's . . . that's got nothing to do with the '90s. That's sort of a superficial, you know, bigotry. That's like ageism or something. It's like if you fought and did good things, we got to give you a gold watch and tell you goodbye.[53]

The political and cultural divide between the pro-Obama, educated, liberal upper-middle class and the less educated, traditional, working-class pro-Clinton supporters became especially evident in the Democratic primary contests. Especially in the Midwest and South, Hillary Clinton's campaign attracted more downscale, less educated, working-class whites and small-town residents.

"Among white voters, socioeconomic status permeates the Obama v. Clinton contest," observed Jay Cost of RealClearPolitics.com. "It seems that one's inclination to vote for a candidate does not depend simply upon age and gender, but age and gender in the context of socioeconomic status. These factors interact with one another. . . . White youth are more likely to vote for Obama than white women or men of all ages, but the particular likelihood that a white youth will vote for Obama also depends upon his or her socioeconomic status. Ditto white females." Income and college variables "account for 40 percent of the variation in Obama's share of the white male vote."[54] The heavily boomer white working-class vote was crucially important in "Republican swing states," that Clinton won in 1996 but that John Kerry lost in 2004. In those states, white boomer voters favored Clinton over Obama by 61 percent to 34 percent.[55]

By the November general election, white boomers (aged forty-five to sixty-four in the CNN exit poll classification) voted for McCain over Obama 56 percent to 42 percent, but this margin differed little from other white age groups except for those aged eighteen to twenty-nine, who voted for Obama over McCain, 54 percent to 44 percent. (About 90 percent of blacks in all age groups voted for Obama, while Obama received almost two-thirds of the Latino vote—with the curious exception of Latino boomers, who gave Obama a 58 percent majority.)[56] Noncollege "working-class" whites gave McCain the exact same margin as they had given George W. Bush: 58 to 40 percent. College-educated whites voted for McCain, 51 percent to 47 percent. (Obama improved over Kerry's 2004 showing by 3 percent.)[57]

Obama was most strongly favored by both the very poor and the very rich. Voters with incomes below $15,000 gave him a 73 percent to 25 percent margin; voters with incomes from $100,000 to $150,000 slightly favored McCain by 51 percent to 48 percent; voters with incomes above $200,000 gave Obama a relatively strong 52 percent to 46 percent advantage—for Republicans, that represented a 17-point drop in support from 2004. (In a postelection poll by National Journal/Heartland Institute, Obama registered unusually high approval levels among several traditionally Republican-leaning high-status occupational groups: 48 percent of the self-employed and 55 percent from college-educated "knowledge workers" such as consultants, engineers, and lawyers.)[58]

These race, class, education, and marital status splits in boomer voting patterns will likely remain. Indeed, the drift of the white working class away from Democrats worried Democratic strategists planning for the 2010 and 2012 elections.[59] Especially via the Tea Party movement (discussed below), middle- and working-class white boomers—including large numbers of small-business and self-employed Americans—appear to have formed the core of an antigovernment, anti-Obama movement, largely among Republicans and Independents. Conversely, the pro-Obama voting coalition has built upon large segments of upper-middle-class professionals, as well as among unmarried women, Latinos, and African Americans (the latter groups now constitute 43 percent of the electorate) and, of course, voters under age thirty.[60]

But the most remarkable age power story was *youth power*. Under-thirty voters were very visibly active in Obama's campaign and gave him a decisive 2–1 majority. If only voters under thirty had voted, Obama would have won 481 Electoral College votes to McCain's 57. But the stability and staying power of this "Generation Obama" remains in doubt.

MILLENNIALS RISING? (NOT YET)

Early in the 2008 primaries, the *New York Times* reporter Katherine Q. Seelye marveled that "age has been one of the most consistent indicators of how someone might vote—more than sex, more than income, more than education. Only race is a stronger predictor of voting than age, and then only if a voter is black, not if he or she is white."[61] This was true throughout the election. The postelection analysis of NBC's Chuck Todd and Sheldon Gawiser offered the understatement that "this year the gap between young and old increased a lot."[62]

"Younger voters," the political scientist Patrick Fisher has observed, "tend to be more liberal and more supportive of Democratic candidates than other age groups." Younger voters are generally more favorable toward activist government and more supportive of spending for both public schools and child care. They are as likely as senior voters to favor increased spending for Social Security, but they are also more favorable to Social Security reform. Fisher concluded that strong age group differences are rooted in different generational value systems. "Younger voters put less of an emphasis on "traditional values." However, Fisher warns that "the partisan polarization in the United States is even greater among younger Americans than it is for the nation as a whole," especially by state and by region.[63]

Millennial Makeover authors Morley Winograd and Michael Hais also find that these children of the boomers differ from their parents and other generations in that they are more practical, civic-minded, optimistic, diverse, and embedded in social networks and groups, as well as more globally and internationally oriented. They are more favorably disposed to government and have almost a 2-to-1 identification with the Democratic Party. Indeed, their defection from Republican ranks is "aging" the GOP's demographic profile: in 1997, 28 percent of GOP voters were over age fifty-five; by 2007, 41 percent were.[64] This, in turn, is driving a generational divide in terms of the different issues emphasized by the two parties. The GOP has highly ranked issues of taxation, national security, immigration, and terrorism. Democrats have been focused more on economic security and inequality, the Iraq War, the environment, and Social Security and Medicare.[65] The latter entitlements, of course, are growing nearer and dearer on a daily basis for aging baby boomers.

Aging boomers hardly seemed threatened by the power of under-thirty voters. (There were many anecdotal stories of adult children convincing boomer parents to vote for Obama.) Indeed, they had little to fear. The Obama-driven youth power movement, reborn after the election as "Organizing for America," proved to be disorganized and ineffectual at promoting the Obama agenda, especially during the 2009–10 congressional health care battles.

Younger voters' infatuation with Obama was ebbing by 2010. The *New York Times* columnist Thomas Friedman wryly observed: "The most striking feature of Barack Obama's campaign for the presidency was the amazing, young, Internet-enabled, grass-roots movement he mobilized to get elected. The most striking feature of Obama's presidency a year later is how thoroughly that movement has disappeared."[66] (A Gallup poll conducted in midsummer 2010 found that Obama's approval rating among those aged eighteen to twenty-nine years had fallen from 65 percent to 54 percent—an 11 percent drop compared to an 8 percent drop among all respondents from 53 percent to 46 percent).[67]

By the 2010 midterm elections Democratic tacticians were belatedly trying to revive the enthusiasm of these youth-based voting brigades. *New York Times* savvy political writer Matt Bai cynically suggested that the midterms were "a test for the real ground game" and that the true remobilization goal was the 2012 presidential campaign.[68] But Democrats were scurrying to energize their youth-women-minorities base for another reason: to counter the rising influence of the Tea Party movement, driven, to a large extent by white, aging baby boomers.[69]

BOOMERS' TEA PARTY TENSIONS: "I WANT SMALLER GOVERNMENT AND MY SOCIAL SECURITY"

The origins of the still amorphous Tea Party movement lie primarily in strong antitax, anti–big government economic reactions against federal government "bailouts" of major corporations and against government "overreach" on health care reform. As a rebellion against "ruling class" efforts to collude and "manage" national problems, the Tea Party's economic populism is clearly a byproduct of the class/political/cultural antagonism discussed above. However, one source of tension within the movement is the desire by some to add conservative religious and social concerns into the movement's agenda. Another, less noticed, source of tension is the tacit acceptance of traditional Social Security and Medicare by its age fifty-plus foot soldiers versus the hard-line libertarian ideology of its younger theoreticians who want to radically restructure such programs.[70]

As mentioned in the previous chapter, the national Tea Party movement has political roots in California's antitax, antigovernment populism that first crystallized in the 1978 "taxpayer revolt" with the successful tax-cutting ballot initiative Proposition 13. Recent data indicate that its sociological base is much the same: overwhelmingly white, middle and working class, and middle-aged or older.

A 2010 Pew report on escalating government mistrust contained an entire section on the Tea Party movement. Though the Tea Party movement has been difficult to study because of its fluid and disorganized structure, the Pew Center's demographic analysis of attitudes toward the Tea Party reinforced a subsequent *New York Times/* CBS News poll's findings of self-identified Tea Party supporters: they are overwhelmingly white and over age fifty—very much a baby boomer phenomenon.[71]

Nearly 30 percent of those responding to the Pew Center's query were unaware of the Tea Party or had no opinion of it. Among those who were aware of the new movement, age, gender, party, and race affected opinions. Strong agreement with the Tea Party agenda increased with age: 33 percent of those over age sixty-five agreed with the movement's agenda compared to 31 percent of the boomer demographic and only 9 percent of those aged eighteen to twenty-nine. Thirty-six percent of men over age fifty were in agreement with the Tea Party but only 14 percent of women aged eighteen to forty-nine. Twenty-eight percent of whites were in agreement compared to 17 percent of Hispanics and 7 percent of blacks. The highest levels of agreement were among Republican college graduates, at 58 percent; Republicans over age fifty, at 54 percent; conservative Republicans, at 53 percent; and Republican men, at 48 percent. (Older, conservative male Republicans are overwhelmingly white.)[72]

A 2010 *New York Times*/CBS poll found similar patterns among self-identified Tea Party supporters: "The 18 percent of Americans who identify themselves as Tea Party supporters tend to be Republican, white, male, married and older than 45." Specifically, 89 percent were white, 59 percent were male, 46 percent were baby boomers (age forty-five to sixty-four), and another 29 percent were over age sixty-four. Fifty-four percent identified as Republican, 36 percent as Independent; 37 percent had a college degree or higher, while 33 percent indicated "some college"; 56 percent earned more than $50,000; 70 percent were married.[73]

The most remarkable aspect of the *Times*/CBS study was reporters' follow-up questions in response to a glaring contradiction: despite the fierce antigovernment, antitax rhetoric, 62 percent of Tea Party identifiers agreed that Social Security and Medicare benefits were "worth the costs." Some justified their current or potential benefits in terms of having paid into the systems. But a sixty-two-year-old baby boomer pondered the contradiction: "Maybe I don't want smaller government. I guess I want smaller government and my Social Security. . . . I didn't look at it from the perspective of losing things I need. I think I've changed my mind."[74]

Aging boomers in the Tea Party and other political venues will be forced to reconsider contradictory commitments to small government and to the old-age entitlements upon which a majority of boomers will be heavily dependent. As their job security, retirement savings, and housing values have dwindled or stagnated during the worst recession since the 1930s, Social Security and Medicare increasingly appear to be the ultimate retirement lifeboats in the unpredictable financial storms of global capitalism. And the only long-standing, reliable guardian of these entitlements is AARP.

But can AARP unite, or at least harness, the wide range of political responses to such issues by a divided boomer generation—especially in the wake of a demoralizing recession and after years of generational infighting?

CHAPTER FOUR

Crash Landing for a
Self-Critical Generation

We baby boomers in America and Western Europe were
raised to believe there really was a Tooth Fairy, whose
magic would allow conservatives to cut taxes without
cutting services and liberals to expand services without
raising taxes. The Tooth Fairy did it by printing money,
by bogus accounting and by deluding us into thinking that
by borrowing from China or Germany, or against our
rising home values, or by creating exotic financial
instruments to trade with each other, we were actually
creating wealth.
—Thomas J. Friedman (2010)

On September 29, 2008, the closing bell at the New York Stock Exchange
began ringing a full minute early. Scattered boos arose from the floor
as exhausted traders were frantically executing a torrent of last-minute
sell orders. Indeed, so great was the volume of "sell at close" orders
from mutual funds that the final, frightening record one-day point loss
of 777 off the Dow Jones Industrial Average didn't fully register until
several minutes after the official end of trading. The plunge was largely
a reaction by professional stock traders to the failure of the House of
Representatives to vote for a seven-hundred-billion-dollar "bailout"
bill designed to address what U.S. Treasury secretary Hank Paulson
and many other financial experts characterized as the nation's most

dangerous financial situation since the 1929 crash. And worse was yet to come.

In the first ten days of October, the Dow lost 2,300 points, declining by more than 40 percent from its all-time high one year earlier. Fifty-five billion dollars had been withdrawn from mutual funds—much of it from 401(k) accounts. The week of October 6 was deemed the worst in Wall Street history. It was followed on October 15 by the second-worst one-day percentage plunge in the Dow since the 1987 crash. By the end of September 2008, the value of the Standard and Poor's stock index of the five hundred largest companies had been basically flat for more than a decade. By mid-November, two trillion dollars had been lost from 401(k) and IRA plans in a mere fifteen months; another two trillion had vanished from company-defined benefit plans; and the average 401(k) had lost 25 percent.[1] The year 2008 would be the worst in stock market history.

The stock market meltdowns vividly illustrated Jacob Hacker's *Risk Shift* warnings about the inherent instability of individually managed 401(k) retirement accounts. Aging boomers' sense of vulnerability had also been "driven home" literally for nearly a year by a more gradual, but nonetheless devastating, deflating residential real estate bubble.

The stock market crash and the evolving "Great Recession" also fanned resentment of private-sector workers toward those in public sector. Private-sector jobs and pensions have proved far more vulnerable than those in government. As I will discuss in greater detail later in this chapter, the longer and more severe the recession, the deeper this "pension envy" is likely to become within baby boomer ranks—and throughout the society as a whole.

The economic downturn also revived the specter of generational conflict via intensified focus on doomsday prophecies about Social Security and Medicare deficits. "A Darker Future for Us," trumpeted a *Newsweek* cover story showcasing AARP foe Robert Samuelson's forthcoming book *The Great Inflation and Its Aftermath.*[2] "Call This a Crisis? Just Wait!" exclaimed the dour David Walker in *Fortune* magazine/

CNN Money.com— who subsequently published his own combination Armageddon-and-redemption volume, *Comeback America: Turning the Country Around and Restoring Fiscal Responsibility* (2009).[3] The economic crises of several European welfare states in 2010 increased critical scrutiny of the American state and local public pensions, Social Security, and Medicare.[4]

Suddenly, retirement and old age were much closer and more precarious than boomers had realized. The financial meltdowns imperiled job security and presumptions of high growth rates of retirement accounts. Boomers' center-stage political status was eclipsed by the successful presidential campaign of self-advertised "postboomer" Barack Obama and his fervent Millennial Generation supporters. In millions of conversations, from water coolers and employee lounges to the Web and the Internet, millions of newly anxious, aging boomers shared worries about job security, retirement, and political hopes and fears—all magnified by 24/7 cable television and the Internet.

During the summer of 2008, workforce expert Carleen MacKay sensed mixed signals from her largely boomer seminar and workshop audiences. On the one hand, she was encouraged that "more employers—and a greater variety of them—are applying for AARP's 'best employers' list. There's a greater appreciation of boomers' education, experience, and institutional memory." On the other hand, employers seemed more interested in retaining aging boomers on a part-time basis rather than full time. As for boomers themselves, especially those unemployed in hard-hit areas like California, MacKay ominously observed, "People are starting to panic. There is no end in sight to foreclosures. I believe absolutely that this recession is going to be a long haul."

By early 2009, an AARP survey of Americans over age forty-five found that 31 percent feared losing a job and that an identical 31 percent feared losing health insurance.[5] Many boomers responded to retirement account and real estate losses by postponing planned retirement dates—if they could keep their jobs.

Busted boomers were *not* necessarily portrayed with great empathy in major news media forums—especially as boomer divisions deepened between supporters of Hillary Clinton and Barack Obama during the long Democratic primaries. The boomer generation was bashed—often by boomers themselves—either as greedy, irresponsible, self-centered "yuppies" or as working- and-lower-middle-class "Tea Party" reactionaries who feared and resented demographic and economic change.

But boomers had reason to be fearful. As discussed in chapter 2, at least 40 percent had been financially ill prepared for retirement *before* the stock market meltdown and deep recession. The recession, stock market swoon, and real estate bust further devalued boomers' two most important retirement assets—their homes and their individual 401(k) retirement accounts heavily invested in stocks and mutual funds.

"The retirement outlook for a large segment of the baby boomer cohort is grim," observed Century Foundation researchers Greg Anrig and Millie Parekh. "In general, they will be more reliant on Social Security and other government protections than imagined just a few short years ago."[6]

CRASH LANDING: SURVIVORS AND CASUALTIES

The bursting real estate bubble, the 2008 stock market crash, and the resulting Great Recession have severely tested aging boomers' abiding faith that there's always one more tomorrow. They were no longer changing society; instead, society was changing them.

Some boomers fared better than others. Most of those who continued to invest in 401(k)s largely recouped their losses, aided by a major stock market rebound in 2009. And some economic simulation models suggest that retirement income from stock market assets for most boomers is likely much smaller than that provided by Social Security. Memories of the crash as a near-death financial experience may linger, but many boomers began to regain their sense of optimism and can-do individualism as steep rises in unemployment and declines in residential real estate values both began to level off in the first half of 2010.

Boomers and other 401(k) participants experienced a rocky retirement account ride from end of the dot-com bust in 2003 through the year of the major stock market crash in 2008. A 2008 Boston College Center for Retirement Research study estimated that the autumn stock market crash erased $2 trillion in 401(k) and IRA accounts and $1.9 trillion more in defined benefit plans. Another $3.6 trillion in household nonpension stocks and mutual funds had melted away.[7] As mentioned in the previous chapter, the number of Older and Younger Boomers "at risk" for having insufficient retirement financial resources (not including probable health care expenses) rose from 35 percent and 44 percent in 2004 to 41 percent and 48 percent, respectively, in 2009.[8]

And yet, somewhat surprisingly, EBRI data show that from 2003 through 2008 all 401(k) age groups who kept making retirement contributions experienced gains for the five-year period (tables 3 and 4). In 2008, those participants with the highest account balances lost somewhat more than those with lower account balances—they had the most to lose. Those in their fifties (Older Boomers) had an average account balance of $79,627 in 2003, with steady annual increases to a high of $148,043 in 2007, followed by a drop of 23.6 percent in 2008 to $113,070—but with an overall gain for the five-year period of 42 percent. Within this age category there were considerable variations by job tenure. Those with thirty years or more on the job had an average account balance of $121,514 in 2003 that rose to a high of $201,302 in 2007 and fell 22.8 percent to $155,309 in 2008—an overall gain during those years of 27.8 percent. Those with the least job tenure (two to five years) had an average account balance of $19,952 in 2003 that rose to a high of $70,177 in 2007, followed by a drop of 18.7 percent to $57,050 in 2008—but an impressive five-year gain of 185.9 percent.[9] (Other EBRI data in this report reveal that the average account balance for all 401(k) accounts rose from $61,106 in 2003 to $114,337 in 2007 and fell to $85,513 in 2008. Median account balances were distressingly low: $25,000 in 2003, $57,000 in 2007, and $43,700 in 2008.)[10]

By the end of 2009, most 401(k) participants who continued monthly contributions were rewarded with a major stock market rebound. Among those aged fifty-five to sixty-four, 401(k) investors with the shortest job tenure actually gained 46.7 percent; those with ten to nineteen years of tenure gained 2.2 percent, while those with twenty to twenty-nine years of tenure lost 2.9 percent. (For those aged forty-five to fifty-four, the corresponding figures were 54.9 percent, 3.1 percent, and −1.8 percent.)[11] Thus a retirement risk model used by EBRI economists since 2003 showed higher percentages of Older and Younger Boomers prepared for retirement in 2010. In 2003, 59.2 percent of Older Boomers were at risk of having insufficient funds to pay for basic retirement costs; by 2010, the figure was 47.2 percent. The corresponding figures for Younger Boomers were 54.7 percent and 43.7 percent. Pre-retirement income strongly structured retirement risk. For example, only 20 percent of Older Boomers in the highest income quartile were at risk for having insufficient retirement funds, versus nearly 80 percent of those in the lowest income quartile.[12]

Paradoxically, though news media attention has focused upon the investment losses of Older Boomers—who have a shorter time span to recoup their losses—the stock markets may ultimately favor them with higher return rates than those obtainable by subsequent generations. The economists Alicia Munnell and Jean-Pierre Aubry found that a hypothetical Older Boomer who had steadily invested in a stock market fund geared to the Standard and Poor's Index since age thirty could have reaped a lifetime annual return rate (through 2009) of 12.4 percent, compared to Younger Boomers' 10.3 percent or Generation X's 8.0 percent. The reason: Older Boomers had the chance to invest during the go-go growth decades of the 1980s and 1990s—eras largely missed by younger investors.[13]

TABLE 3

Average Account Balances among 401(k) Participants Present from Year-End 2003 through Year-End 2008, by Participant Age and Tenure

Age Group	Tenure (years)	2003	2004	2005	2006	2007	2008
20s	All	$4,579	$8,286	$12,335	$17,568	$22,851	$18,598
	>2–5	$1,594	$5,634	$10,315	$15,999	$21,825	$17,909
	>5–10	$4,776	$8,491	$12,498	$17,735	$23,024	$18,799
30s	All	$19,316	$26,660	$33,816	$43,915	$53,464	$39,883
	>2–5	$6,210	$13,630	$21,547	$31,456	$41,072	$32,336
	>5–10	$14,289	$21,320	$28,381	$37,911	$47,121	$35,789
	>10–20	$27,792	$35,616	$42,881	$53,881	$63,989	$46,629
40s	All	$48,092	$59,727	$70,115	$86,165	$100,744	$74,148
	>2–5	$13,240	$23,320	$33,471	$46,380	$58,732	$45,960
	>5–10	$22,002	$31,270	$40,337	$52,627	$64,286	$48,848
	>10–20	$49,714	$61,158	$71,347	$87,298	$101,782	$73,976
	>20–30	$87,148	$103,135	$116,162	$138,666	$158,358	$116,064
50s	All	$79,627	$95,049	$107,945	$129,073	$148,043	$113,070
	>2–5	$19,952	$31,122	$41,772	$56,042	$70,177	$57,050
	>5–10	$25,434	$35,399	$45,165	$58,373	$71,096	$56,282
	>10–20	$56,952	$69,714	$80,981	$98,397	$114,090	$86,560
	>20–30	$120,920	$141,472	$158,138	$186,832	$212,560	$160,521
	>30	$121,514	$140,254	$153,928	$179,468	$201,302	$155,309
60s	All	$105,663	$120,541	$130,743	$148,882	$162,290	$125,052
	>2–5	$28,990	$40,279	$50,635	$64,075	$77,142	$62,956
	>5–10	$27,535	$37,533	$46,961	$59,262	$70,201	$55,831
	>10–20	$61,052	$73,844	$84,527	$100,068	$112,393	$85,587
	>20–30	$128,691	$147,324	$160,313	$182,439	$197,671	$150,787
	>30	$171,417	$188,257	$196,590	$217,459	$231,880	$179,573
All	All	$61,106	$73,253	$83,441	$99,864	$114,337	$86,513

SOURCE: Jack VanDerhei, Sarah Holden, and Luis Alonso, "401(k) Plan Asset Allocation, Account Balances, and Loan Activity in 2008," *Employee Benefit Research Institute Issue Brief,* no. 335 (October 2009), 12. (Tabulations from EBRI/ICI Participant-Directed Retirement Plan Data Collection Project.)

NOTE: The analysis is based on a sample of six million participants with account balances at the end of each year from 2003 through 2008. Age and tenure groups are based on participant age and tenure at year-end 2008.

TABLE 4

Percent Change in Average Account Balances among 401(k) Participants Present from Year-End 2003 through Year-End 2008, by Participant Age and Tenure

Age Group	Tenure (years)	2003–4	2004–5	2005–6	2006–7	2007–8	2003–8
20s	All	81.0%	48.9%	42.4%	30.1%	−18.6%	306.2%
	>2–5	253.5%	83.1%	55.1%	36.4%	−17.9%	1023.5%
	>5–10	77.8%	47.2%	41.9%	29.8%	−18.4%	293.2%
30s	All	38.0%	26.8%	29.9%	21.7%	−25.4%	106.5%
	>2–5	119.5%	58.1%	46.0%	30.6%	−21.3%	420.7%
	>5–10	49.2%	33.1%	33.6%	24.3%	−24.0%	150.5%
	>10–20	28.2%	20.4%	25.7%	18.8%	−27.1%	67.8%
40s	All	24.2%	17.4%	22.9%	16.9%	−26.4%	54.2%
	>2–5	76.1%	43.5%	38.6%	26.6%	−21.7%	247.1%
	>5–10	42.1%	29.0%	30.5%	22.2%	−24.0%	122.0%
	>10–20	23.0%	16.7%	22.4%	16.6%	−27.3%	48.8%
	>20–30	18.3%	12.6%	19.4%	14.2%	−26.7%	33.2%
50s	All	19.4%	13.6%	19.6%	14.7%	−23.6%	42.0%
	>2–5	56.0%	34.2%	34.2%	25.2%	−18.7%	185.9%
	>5–10	39.2%	27.6%	29.2%	21.8%	−20.8%	121.3%
	>10–20	22.4%	16.2%	21.5%	15.9%	−24.1%	52.0%
	>20–30	17.0%	11.8%	18.1%	13.8%	−24.5%	32.7%
	>30	15.4%	9.7%	16.6%	12.2%	−22.8%	27.8%
60s	All	14.1%	8.5%	13.9%	9.0%	−22.9%	18.3%
	>2–5	38.9%	25.7%	26.5%	20.4%	−18.4%	117.2%
	>5–10	36.3%	25.1%	26.2%	18.5%	−20.5%	102.8%
	>10–20	21.0%	14.5%	18.4%	12.3%	−23.9%	40.2%
	>20–30	14.5%	8.8%	13.8%	8.3%	−23.7%	17.2%
	>30	9.8%	4.4%	10.6%	6.6%	−22.6%	4.8%
All	All	19.9%	13.9%	19.7%	14.5%	−24.3%	41.6%

SOURCE: Jack VanDerhei, Sarah Holden, and Luis Alonso, "401(k) Plan Asset Allocation, Account Balances, and Loan Activity in 2008," *Employee Benefit Research Institute Issue Brief,* no. 335 (October 2009), 12. (Tabulations from EBRI/ICI Participant-Directed Retirement Plan Data Collection Project.)

NOTE: The analysis is based on a sample of six million participants with account balances at the end of each year from 2003 through 2008. Age and tenure groups are based on participant age and tenure at year-end 2008.

Real Estate Roulette

Of somewhat greater concern to millions of both Older and Younger Boomers was the collapse in the price of housing, for many their primary asset. Depending upon geographical region, average home price losses equaled stock market declines. During 2008, for the largest twenty cities, the Case Shiller real estate index fell by a record 19 percent in one year. On the East and West Coasts and in Florida the situation was worse. In many areas of California, property values fell more than 50 percent; in California's vast "Inland Empire" area just east of Los Angeles, twenty years of real estate price gains were wiped out.[14] In New York City, the median price of a house declined 19 percent, and a major bank predicted further declines as more residents lost jobs.[15]

"As a result of the plunge in house prices, many baby boomers now have little or no equity in their home," a 2009 Center for Economic and Policy Research study concluded. From 2004 to 2009, Older Boomers (aged fifty-five to sixty-four) saw their median household net worth fall by almost 50 percent, from $315,400 to $159,800; for Younger Boomers (aged forty-five to fifty-four), net worth fell by more than 45 percent, from $172,400 to $94,000. The center estimated that perhaps 15 percent of Older Boomers and 30 percent of Younger Boomers were "underwater"—their mortgage was worth more than the market value of their home.[16] (A surprisingly large number of boomers' older siblings had also been sucked into the real estate maelstrom: by 2007, 43 percent of Americans aged sixty-five to seventy-two had mortgages—up from 18 percent in 1992.)[17]

In the fourth quarter of 2008, according to a Federal Reserve report, the average net worth of American households declined a record 9 percent, the steepest quarterly decline in fifty years. This was a 20 percent fall from its all-time high of $64.36 trillion in the second quarter of 2007. (The median net worth decline was 18 percent.)[18] By the end of 2009, household net worth was still down nearly 17 percent.[19]

The impact of the decline fell disproportionately upon wealthiest households and those between the ages of fifty-five and sixty-four—primarily the Older Boomers.[20] Baby boomers responded to these losses by cutting their spending by almost one-third. According to a Gallup poll, average daily spending fell from an average of $98 in 2008 to $64 in 2009—a decline greater than any other age group.[21]

The Continuing Importance of Social Security

Some economic models suggest that the impact of the stock market plunge may have been overstated. First, nearly one-third of boomers had failed to invest in the market at all and therefore had little or nothing to lose in the 2008 plunge. About 37 percent of Americans born between 1941 and 1965 owned no stocks when the market crashed (though those with traditional pensions were indirect stockholders). Second, contrary to studies suggesting that the stock market plunge would adversely affect large numbers of aging boomers, an Urban Institute retirement income simulation model estimated that "income from assets will account for a small share of retirement income, even for those with stocks. For most retirees, Social Security provides the majority of income."[22]

Economists at the National Bureau of Economic Research concurred. Their simulation model suggested that the declining values of independent retirement accounts and home values might have little effect on retirement decisions of Older Boomers because they had only 15.2 percent of their wealth in stocks via independent retirement accounts (IRAs or 401(k)s). And these amounts were dwarfed by the value of their Social Security accounts.[23]

However, massive layoffs during the Great Recession likely led many more boomers to "cash in early" on Social Security, diminishing the value of those accounts—as well as their lifetime benefits. Claiming early Social Security retirement benefits at age sixty-two, instead of waiting until the full benefits threshold of age sixty-six, reduces

monthly payouts by 25 percent. Millions of boomers have been choos-
ing this option. The number of retired workers who began collecting
Social Security in fiscal 2009 jumped nearly 19 percent; the total number of applications (including disability) rose 23 percent, handily beating a 15 percent projected increase. Much of the 8 percent additional
rise was attributed to rising unemployment among the 3.4 million baby
boomers turning sixty-two in 2009.[24] The surge in filings was so great
that, in combination with declining payroll taxes, Social Security was
projected to be in deficit in 2010—for the first time since 1975 (the year
of another major recession).[25] Before the 2008 economic turmoil, at least
half of boomers were expected to file for Social Security at age sixty-
two; a full 75 percent are still thought likely to file sometime before
qualifying for full benefit levels at age sixty-six.[26]

Employers slashed over 8.4 million jobs during the Great Recession.
The *USA Today* reporter Dennis Cauchon concluded that "baby boomers . . . have been hit particularly hard." While the number of jobless
in the general population doubled, unemployment among those aged
fifty-five to sixty-four tripled.[27] Unemployment rates for workers forty-
five and older soared to their highest level since 1948.[28] For men over
age fifty-five, the unemployment rate was a record 7.7 percent—-before
starting a very slow decline throughout 2010. While workers over forty-
five generally have lower unemployment rates than the younger jobless,
a higher proportion of older workers are out of work for more than six
months, and they are more likely to earn less in new jobs.[29] Not surprisingly, an ABC News Poll found that those aged forty-five to fifty-
four were the most pessimistic age group about future job security and
retirement prospects.[30]

Beneath these general unemployment statistics was another dimen-
sion of the potent class and educational divide among boomers discussed in the previous chapter: lower levels of class and education
increase prospects for involuntary, early retirement.

The economists Courtney Coile and Philip Levine estimate that the
majority of the 378,000 workers pushed into retirement as the result of

the recession are more likely to have less education and lower income and asset levels, so that they are (necessarily) more sensitive to unemployment and labor market conditions. Conversely, unemployed persons with higher incomes, assets, and educational levels are better prepared to endure short or medium-length periods of unemployment without having to turn to Social Security. They also may be better able to regain employment and work longer. And they are more attuned to stock market conditions in determining their retirement outlooks.[31]

RECOVERY OR STAGNATION?

In September 2010, the National Bureau of Economic Research, reviewing months of national productivity data, declared that the Great Recession had officially ended in June 2009. Many Americans, still coping with a national unemployment rate approaching 10 percent, were skeptical. Yet by early 2010, the EBRI Retirement Confidence Survey detected a slight uptick in retirement confidence: 16 percent of respondents were "very confident" of a secure retirement—up from the record low of 13 percent in 2009. Twenty-nine percent were very confident about being able to pay for basic retirement expenses—up from 25 percent in 2009 but down from a significantly higher 34 percent in 2008.[32] (A Watson-Wyatt 2009 survey found—not surprisingly—that 55 percent of those with lifetime defined-benefit pensions were "very confident" about near-term retirement security compared to 38 percent of those with only defined-contribution plans.)[33]

The Natural Marketing Institute consultant Steve French also sensed a tentative rebound of boomer self-confidence measured via the institute's ongoing database. Forty percent of boomer respondents claimed to be "on target" with retirement planning investments—a return to precrash levels. Responsibility and self-reliance measures remained strong: 85 percent of boomers responded that they would have to rely on "myself" to maintain retirement independence. The percentage agreeing that they would need to rely on government "a lot" or "somewhat" in retirement declined from 59 percent in 2006 to 48 percent in 2010. But these expectations of retirement self-reliance were somewhat compromised by findings that a majority of boomer respondents also appeared willfully ignorant about their own retirement planning—admitting that they were "somewhat scared" or "didn't know" about whether they were saving enough for retirement. (Indeed, 18 percent of boomers in French's sample had no retirement savings at all.)[34]

Leaders in the financial services industry felt vindicated by the revival of investor confidence and fortunes. By December 31, 2009, retirement accounts assets rose 18 percent over the previous year to $9.3 trillion.[35] Calls for government intervention and reform of individual retirement accounts became less urgent. "Savers are sticking with a 401(k) plan," declared Vanguard Mutual Funds chair emeritus John Brennan. Indeed, a 2009 Vanguard study found that 60 percent of Vanguard's individual retirement investors had account balances that had held steady or increased.[36] Brennan and Paul Stevens, president of the Investment Company Institute, were also pleased to cite results of an ICI survey of American households: 90 percent had a favorable view of 401(k) plans, and 96 percent did not want government regulations to limit individual choices.[37] (This was welcome ammunition to use against a possible push by the Obama administration to encourage workers to convert more volatile stock-market-based individual retirement accounts into annuity policies.)[38]

But by mid-2010 consumer confidence began to sink once again. A front-page *Wall Street Journal* report documented continued high outflows from stock mutual funds and concluded that "ordinary investors are returning to the cautious mentality they developed during the 1970s. That was the last extended period of stock weakness, after which it took many people a decade or more to get comfortable with stocks again."[39]

The Great Recession was altering Americans' behavior and outlook. By mid-2010, a Pew Research Center survey of three thousand

American adults found that 55 percent had experienced a cut in pay, a reduction in hours, or involuntary part-time work. Sixty percent had cut back spending. Though the young were hardest hit in terms of unemployment, boomers and those over sixty-five tended to perceive greater impact. Fifty-seven percent of respondents aged fifty to sixty-four (boomers) reported their financial situation was worse today than before the recession (compared to 48 percent of those aged thirty to forty-nine and 42 percent of those over age sixty-five). Twenty-seven percent of those aged fifty to sixty-four and 29 percent of those over sixty-five thought that the financial situation in the coming year would get worse—compared to a mere 8 percent of those aged eighteen to twenty-nine and 14 percent of those aged thirty to forty-nine. Twenty-one percent of those over age fifty thought the recession had wrought permanent changes in the economy compared to 13 percent of those aged eighteen to twenty-four and 16 percent of those aged twenty-five to forty-nine.[40] Noting that respondents earning over $75,000 were also among the most pessimistic, the *Washington Post* economist Robert Samuelson concluded that "one legacy of the Great Recession is that insecurity and uncertainty have gone upscale. . . . The Great Recession, though jarring to almost everyone, has been most disruptive and disillusioning to those who were previously the most protected."[41] Aging boomers were under pressure as never before to increase their rate of savings and to keep working—if they could keep their jobs.

GREAT EXPECTATIONS, GRIM REALITIES: WORKING LONGER, SAVING MORE?

For at least a decade, many aging boomers have indicated that they intend to make up for inadequate retirement savings by working longer and saving more.[42] Quantitative models developed prior to the 2008 stock market meltdown by Munnell et al. and by Farrell et al. (McKinsey Global Institute) encourage this strategy. According to the latter, "Our analysis shows that enabling the Boomers to work later in life would significantly benefit both individual households and the broader economy. By increasing the median retirement age by about two years—from 62.6 today to 64.1 by 2015—the share of unprepared Boomer households could be halved from 62 percent to 31 percent. And the additional workers would boost real GDP growth."[43]

More boomers are listening. "Among workers age 50 to 61 fully 63% say they might have to push back their expected retirement because of current economic conditions," according to a Pew Research Center report. A majority of older workers claim they remain on the job because they want to. Of those over age sixty-five who are working, 54 percent do so because they want to work; just 17 percent claim they work only for the paycheck.[44] Yet work satisfaction levels have dropped steeply during the past twenty years, especially among older workers. According to a Conference Board report, 70.8 percent of workers over sixty-five were satisfied with their work in 1987; by 2009, only 43.4 percent were. (In the age fifty-five to sixty-four category—which includes most of today's Older Boomers—the drop from 1987 to 2009 was from 59.3 to 45.6 percent.)[45]

The 2000–2010 decade has taken a toll on American workers' confidence regarding retirement. In 2000, 74 percent of workers were confident or somewhat confident that they would have enough money to live comfortably in retirement; by 2010, the figure was 64 percent. In 2000, 84 percent were confident in having enough money to meet basic expenses; in 2010, the figure was 75 percent. And in 2000, 66 percent were confident they would be able to pay for medical expenses in retirement; by 2010, that number had dropped to 49 percent.[46]

Dreams of early retirement have largely faded. In 2000, 12 percent of workers over age fifty-five thought they would retire before age sixty; by 2010, the figure was 2 percent. (For those in the age forty-five to fifty-four bracket, the corresponding figures were 24 percent and 6 percent.) Instead, more Americans over age forty-five plan to work longer: in 2000 only 20 percent of workers over age fifty-five thought they would work until age sixty-six or older; by 2010, the percentage doubled to 42 percent. (For those in the forty-five to fifty-four bracket, the corresponding figures were 18 and 33 percent.)[47]

Alas, research reveals a substantial gap between optimistic intentions to work beyond or to the age of sixty-five and actual outcomes. For example, nearly half of respondents (46 percent) in the AARP survey entitled "Boomers Turning 60" were *already* retired.[48] Surveys by other organizations indicate that such large-scale retirements may not have been entirely voluntary. A 2006 McKinsey and Company survey found that 40 percent of preretired boomers planned to work beyond age sixty-five but that only 13 percent of current retirees had actually done so. Nearly 40 percent of current retirees had been forced to retire primarily because of health reasons (47 percent) or because of job loss (44 percent).[49]

Similar findings were obtained in a more recent EBRI study. Half of preretired workers intended to retire at age sixty-five or later, but only 28 percent of current retirees had done so. Conversely, only 28 percent of preretirees planned to retire before age sixty-five, but 62 percent of actual retirees left work before that age. Those who retired early cited health problems or disability (24 percent), employment changes such as downsizing or employer closure (34 percent), or responsibilities of caring for a spouse or family members (18 percent).[50] As mentioned above, the unexpectedly large number of early Social Security filings in 2009 suggests a continuing or even widening gap between aging boomers' actual retirement age and their willingness or ability to work longer or, for those who lose jobs, to gain re-employment.

Then there is the question of age bias and whether employers want to retain aging workers. Indeed, even before the 2008 economic turmoil, Alicia Munnell and the *Wall Street Journal*'s David Wessel had doubts: "The image of loyal companies retaining scarce, seasoned workers is at odds with reality. Among male workers between 58 and 62, only 44 percent still work for the outfit that employed them at 50, down from 70 percent two decades ago. And even if labor shortages emerge, employers will likely hire younger immigrants, shift work overseas, or deploy labor-saving technology instead of hiring older workers."[51]

The Equal Employment Opportunity Commission reported that age discrimination claims rose 30 percent in 2008,[52] suggesting that, as Julian Mincer reported in the *Wall Street Journal,* "baby boomers have gone from being treasured to, in many cases, terminated."[53] In 2009, *New York Times* "Generation B" reporter Michael Winerip interviewed two dozen boomers at a Manhattan job fair that normally attracted 1,500 college-age job seekers but had ballooned to 5,103—mostly baby boomers seeking reemployment.[54] When he reinterviewed sixteen of them a year later, nine were "still struggling" and only one had found a job that paid more than his old one.[55]

The retirement economic expert Alicia Munnell grew even more pessimistic about many boomers' ability to recoup retirement losses. While still urging older Americans to work longer, she nonetheless admitted: "People who got caught in this downdraft in their fifties simply don't have time to increase their savings by an amount that would be sufficient. Your savings rate would have to be so high that you wouldn't have enough to live on."[56] The noted economist and stock market forecaster Edward Yardeni indicted the whole individual retirement account system: "There's just no way you can really save out of the median income in this country and retire comfortably."[57] He grimly observed that many people who know they're already far behind in building a nest egg for retirement are going to realize that trying to catch up is practically impossible and will simply give up.[58]

A more optimistic scenario for continued employment among highly educated Older Boomers was set forth in a 2010 Metlife report on the retirement prospects of "Early Boomers." As first mentioned in chapter 1, the study found that male boomers aged sixty to sixty-four had the highest college graduation rate (37 percent) of any older or younger generation segment. In addition, 75 percent of Older Boomer women and three-fifths of the men were white-collar workers—an occupational group less vulnerable to layoffs than lower-skilled blue-collar workers. The report's authors predicted that by the time Older Boomers approached age seventy over half of them would still be working—compared to the previous retirement rate of 75 percent by age sixty-five.[59]

Predictions of labor shortages have begun to resurface. For example, Barry Bluestone and Mark Melnick predicted that if the recovery continued, along with current labor and immigration trends, there might be millions of new jobs available, especially in social services, health care, and nonprofit sectors.[60] However, these jobs might be slow to develop.

With such uncertain forecasts and after waves of layoffs by corporations and, by 2010, significant reductions of state and local public employees, many fifty-plus Americans have been pondering the uncertain call of self-employment. How viable a route is that?

Salvation through Self-Employment?

Small business enthusiasts suggest that aging boomers can remedy job and retirement savings loss by becoming independent consultants or entrepreneurs—part of what author Daniel Pink terms "Free Agent Nation."[61] Indeed, according to the Small Business Administration, the number of self-employed people aged fifty-five to sixty-five has soared, climbing 52 percent from 2000 to 2007.[62]

"Boomers Move to Self Employment," *Forbes's* Ashlea Ebeling cheerfully reported. "Rising unemployment reinforces their entrepreneurial bent."[63] Data on small business start-ups and failures are scarce. But boosters for boomer small businesses often point to Kauffman Foundation data suggesting that successful start-ups are as likely to be founded by older as younger Americans—in one survey 18 percent of small business founders were over age fifty-five.[64]

"In the not-too-distant future, older workers who are self employed, independent contractors, or consultants may outnumber older workers in salaried employment," wrote *The Long Baby Boom* author James

Goldsmith.[65] Aging boomers want to work longer, more will be healthy enough to sustain longer careers, and more will be needed to fill projected shortages of skilled workers. The increasing prominence of knowledge workers who work for themselves and the rise in telecommuting bode well for lengthening boomers' working years.[66]

Nearly all small business enthusiasts agree that the major roadblock for would-be boomer entrepreneurs has been affordable health insurance—especially for anyone with a preexisting condition. "The difficulties of health insurance can negate all the benefits of being your own boss," concludes Laura Vanderkam in a recent overview of self-employment statistics.[67] (High health insurance costs are an increasing problem for those who already own small enterprises.)[68]

If the recently enacted Patient Protection and Affordable Care Act reduces insurance costs for individuals and small companies, then the microtrend expert Mark Penn foresees a resurgence of self-employment, a rejuvenated land of entrepreneurs he terms "Boss Nation."[69] But Penn admits that current economic conditions are hardly ideal for self-employment start-ups.

Indeed, data on small business failure are hard to come by, but the risk of failure in the current economic climate is likely high and doubly tragic if retirement funds are funneled into failing small businesses. (Many retirement planners must surely cringe at upbeat news media reports on "the IRA Job Machine," describing how displaced workers are cashing out their retirement savings to start independent ventures.)[70]

However, aging boomers who remain employed in the public sector or in a dwindling number of major corporations still have one huge advantage: defined-benefit pensions that provide lifetime incomes.

Pension Envy

Many boomers will have sources of retirement income other than Social Security and individual retirement accounts. Perhaps half of boomer individuals (through their own employer or their spouse's) will be covered by a defined-benefit pension plan that will theoretically provide lifetime retirement income—if the plan remains financially solvent. Some pension systems are much better and safer than others—especially taxpayer-guaranteed public pension plans. Pension envy could create a potent new divide among aging baby boomers, especially between those who have taxpayer-guaranteed, often relatively generous public pensions, and those with less secure private pensions, unstable private retirement accounts—or none at all.

Fewer than one out of four private-sector workers has a defined benefit pension. But four out of five public-sector workers participate in such plans. Stock market losses and recession have battered both private and public pension funding reserves; but public pensions are legally guaranteed by federal, state, and local government.

Forbes reporter Stephane Fitch was one of the first to contrast private-sector and public-sector retirement disparities. "In private sector America the math leads to the grim prospect of working longer and living poorer. . . . In public sector America things just get better and better. The common presumption is that public servants forgo high wages in exchange for safe jobs and benefits. The reality is they get all three. State and local government workers get paid an average of $25.30 an hour, which is 33 percent higher than the private sector's $19, according to Bureau of Labor Statistics data. Throw in pensions and other benefits and the gap widens to 42 percent."[71]

"One wonders," mused the veteran *Sacramento Bee* columnist Dan Walters, "how long taxpayers, many of whom are seeing reductions in their incomes and watching their 401(k) pension funds wither, will tolerate new taxes or reductions in other spending to prop up public pensions that are much more generous than their own."[72]

Technically, some forty-four million private-sector employees or retirees are covered by defined-benefit plans. Many of these plans were underfunded before the economic turmoil of 2008. But by the end of 2008, Standard and Poor's five hundred largest companies had a combined pension deficit of $376 billion at the end of 2008. (For example, giant Caterpillar Corporation had $10.4 billion in its pension fund at the end of 2007—about seven hundred million dollars less than its obligations. By the end of 2008, those assets were at $2.8 billion. The company hoped to contribute one billion dollars during 2009—and also laid off twenty thousand workers.)[73] By August 2010, the total pension deficit for the Standard and Poor's largest 1,500 companies hit a record high of $506 billion.[74]

Corporations have been reducing pension liabilities by converting defined benefit plans to cash balances and/or defined-contribution—401(k)—systems.[75] The remaining private-sector pensions are theoretically insured by the federal government's Pension Benefit Guaranty Corporation. Alas, that agency's own year-end deficit doubled from $11.2 billion in 2008 to $21.9 billion in 2009. Furthermore, as United Airlines' once highly compensated pilots discovered during that airline's bankruptcy, when company pensions are dumped onto PBGC, the annual benefits may be considerably less than those once promised by the company. (The PBGC maximum annual individual retirement benefit—taken at age sixty-five—is currently $54,000.)[76] For the 22.5 million public-sector workers, the picture is much different. Four out of five public-sector workers are covered by defined-benefit lifetime pensions. Public pension payouts are often calibrated to provide retirement incomes based upon an individual's highest-income years while working. In states with strong public unions, such as California, many police and firefighters can retire in their fifties with nearly 100 percent of their active-duty pay. (If they qualify for disability status, pensioners can make more as retirees than when they were working. This has led to system abuses and scandals—as when the *New York Times* discovered that nearly all career employees of the Long Island Railroad qualified for retirement disability payments.)[77]

The stock market meltdown exposed enormous public pension liabilities just as baby boomers in that sector begin retiring. In 2009, California was paying three billion dollars a year into its pension fund—ten times what it had a decade before.[78] But by mid-June of that same year, the giant California Public Employees' Retirement System (CalPERS) had lost nearly 23 percent of its portfolio value and could cover only 61 percent of future liabilities.[79] Across the country, New York City's pension contributions almost tripled from $1.4 billion in 2002 to $6.3 billion in 2009, and its estimated contributions for 2016 are $10 billion.[80] And even such rapidly escalating payments might prove insufficient.

Adequate levels of funding for state and local government pension liabilities were declining even before the 2008 stock market crash.[81] A 2007 U.S. Government Accountability Office evaluation found that, on the basis of 2006 fiscal year data, most state and local government agencies' pensions were adequately funded. But a 2008 GAO report—still based on year-old data—found that nearly 42 percent of state and local government pension plans were funded at less than the recommended level of 80 percent of liabilities.[82] By the end of fiscal year 2008, a Pew Center on the States report found eight states with only two-thirds (or less) of recommended state pension funding reserves: Connecticut, Illinois, Kansas, Kentucky, Massachusetts, Oklahoma, Rhode Island, and West Virginia.[83] A more recent assessment of 2009 fiscal year data on public pension funding levels by the Boston College Center for Retirement Research found that 58 percent of all public pension plans were below the recommended 80 percent level and warned that "the decline is only the beginning of the bad news that will emerge as the losses are spread over the next several years. . . . Under our most likely scenario, funding rates will decline to 72 percent by 2013."[84]

Funding reserves for most public-sector retiree health plans are even more precarious.[85] Until 2007, lax actuarial standards allowed public officials to overlook this second hidden fiscal time bomb.[86] For example, unfunded retiree health care costs for the Los Angeles Unified School District are estimated by the state legislative analyst's office to range from five billion to ten billion dollars over the next thirty years. At a minimum, the district should be contributing five hundred million dollars a year; instead it has set aside nothing.[87] The state of California will likely pay more than one billion dollars a year for retiree health care costs—perhaps much more. Health benefits for a retired, married state pensioner (and spouse) may eventually cost the state five hundred thousand to one million dollars.[88]

By mid-2010, the ultimate taxpayer bill for this emerging public pension aristocracy was generating so much public and professional alarm that the *New York Times* and the *Wall Street Journal* provided major public pension liability forums on the same day.[89] By the autumn of 2010, a steady drumbeat of grim reports bolstered speculation that the next "sovereign debt crisis" would not come from bankrupt foreign nations such as Greece but from "California, New Jersey, Illinois and Ohio."[90]

By one estimate, California's state and local government unfunded pension liabilities of $325 billion amounted to an individual debt of $22,000 for every California working adult. California governor Arnold Schwarzenegger declared escalating pension costs to be the state's number one policy problem, and a series of editorials and reports in the *Los Angeles Times* increasingly chronicled how several cities and state agencies were struggling to balance rapidly rising pension costs with money for basic public and social services.[91]

As discussed in chapter 2's California case study, public pension battles may trigger age-based politics related to other social divisions: public pensioners are disproportionately white and, increasingly, baby boomers; but the younger population of more ethnically diverse taxpayers, struggling economically and far less likely to participate in defined benefit plans, may resent paying this increasingly expensive eldercare tab.

A SELF-CRITICAL GENERATION

"I don't see how we got from there to here," sighed retirement researcher Mathew Greenwald. His boomer brethren's youthful cultural emphases on self-denial, antimaterialism, and self-directed expression had become proestablishment, promaterialism, and obsession with expensive lifestyles. One year before the 2008 stock market crash, Greenwald warned me that "boomers are *very* economically vulnerable." Millions will reach their retirement years financially unprepared, only to face inevitable entitlement cutbacks. "Boomers will become infuriated," Greenwald predicted; they will try to mobilize political pressure. But they will not be regarded sympathetically. "They'll be told, 'Boomers, you screwed up.'"[92]

Two years later, Greenwald's prediction was illustrated in an e-mail response to National Public Radio's nationally syndicated *Diane Rehm Show* (August 13, 2008). Entitlement critic David Walker (former U.S. controller general and Peter G. Peterson Foundation executive director) had railed against the growth of the national debt and the impending fiscal crises of Social Security and Medicare. Listeners responded.

> MS. REHM: Here's an e-mail from Jane in St. Louis, Missouri. She says, "I'm a thirty-four-year-old mother of two boys. My husband and I are part of Generation X; we do not believe there will be any Social Security or health care benefits through the federal government when we retire. My generation is very angry for the irresponsible spending of the baby boomers. I love my parents and want them taken care of, but I see a future where my generation cuts off the older generation because we won't be able to afford to take care of them and we'll consider it their just deserts as the new generation ages and younger generations come into power and they may find the plastic spoon cut off.
>
> DAVID WALKER: Well, first I think we have to avoid intergenerational conflict if at all possible . . .

But the seeds of conflict within and between generations had already emerged in the Democratic primary contest between archetypal boomer Hillary Rodham Clinton and Barack Obama, the self-styled "postboomer" candidate. As discussed in the previous chapter, rhetoric and votes often reflected the class-cultural divide.

The Clinton-Obama primary battles inspired an industry of both caustic and humorous commentary about boomers' values, lifestyles, and 1960s heritage. The latter was also fueled by media commemorations of the fortieth anniversary of 1968—notably via books such as Tom Brokaw's best-selling *Boom!* (advertised as a 650-page "class reunion" of 1960s leaders). Much of the mass media labeling of boomers—often by boomers themselves—was self-critical if not self-loathing. As aging boomers become older and more vulnerable, the wave of largely unanswered boomer bashing could come back to haunt them.[93]

Boomers Bashing Boomers

Boomers' liberal 1960s heritage—personified in Bill and Hillary Clinton—was almost always unfavorably compared with Obama's brand of postboomer, postracial, and postpartisan liberalism. Most big-name, boomer-aged pundits were enchanted by Obama.[94] Conversely, pundits such as George Will zestfully cast Hillary and Bill Clinton as ambitious, self-centered "generational archetypes." *Newsweek's* Howard Fineman archly concurred: "As always—and for better or worse—Bill Clinton sums up the political persona and aspirations of his generation: the emotional brew of idealism and self-centeredness; the view of public life as a perpetual 'fight' purified to abstraction by the boomers' relative lack of experience on real battlefields."[95]

The Obama campaign offered liberal aging boomers a second chance to revive their 1960s hopes and visions. Peter Feld noted that "the early Boomers for whom the late '60s activism was formative are a small but visible group, now at the peak of its influence. Many of them are politicians, journalists, or donors. For many of them, the wounds of the seminal year of 1968 never healed. . . . As these children of the '60s start to enter their 60s, their sense of unfinished business takes on urgency. Now Obama—seemingly Robert F. Kennedy and the Rev. Martin Luther King rolled into one—offers them a two-for-one redemption of 1968's political assassination of where America left off."[96]

Thus *New York Times* columnist Frank Rich (a boomer) blessed the Obama candidacy's updated liberalism: "Mr. Obama is a liberal, but he is not your boomer parents' liberalism." Obama recognizes "the expiring shelf life" of Clinton-Bush era policies and "never rattles off a Clinton laundry list of big federal programs.... The selling point of Mr. Obama's vision of change is not doctrinaire liberalism or Bush-bashing but an inclusiveness that he believes can start to relieve Washington's gridlock much as it animated his campaign. Some of that inclusiveness is racial, ethnic and generational, in the casual, what's-the-big-deal manner of post-boomer Americans already swimming in our country's rapidly expanding demographic pool."[97]

The nostalgia for 1960s social movements evoked by the Obama campaign and fortieth-anniversary celebrations of 1968 in the mass media incensed conservative commentators—often baby boomers themselves. They invoked the World War II "Greatest Generation" legacy of boomers' parents to scorn their offspring's 1960s heritage.

The Greatest Generation's major mistake was that "it begat the boomers," sneered *Weekly Standard* senior editor William Kristol (a boomer), responding to Tom Brokaw's book *Boom!,* a positive portrait of the 1960s. "The most prominent of the boomers spent their youth scorning those of their compatriots who fought communism, while moralizing and posturing at no cost to themselves. They went on to enjoy the benefits of their parents' labors, sacrificed little, and produced nothing particularly notable. But the boomers were unparalleled when it came to self-glorification."[98]

"Spoiled brat baby boomers!" is conservative talk radio host Rush Limbaugh's stock putdown for his own generation. The baby boomer political analyst Michael Barone grumbled that "for the past 15 years, our politics has been a civil war between two halves of the baby boom generation. . . . And we are tired of it. Most voters would like to move on to something new."[99] And the Hoover Institution classicist Victor Davis Hansen (another baby boomer) joined the self-critical conservative chorus: "What are the baby boomers' collective traits? Like all perpetual adolescents who suffer arrested development, we always want things both ways. . . . Perhaps the greatest trademark of the 1960s cohort was self-congratulation. Baby boomers alone claimed to have brought about changes in civil rights, women's liberation and environmental awareness—as if these were not prior concerns of earlier generations."[100]

Conservatives have tried to utilize lingering resentment of the boomers' 1960s heritage for overtly political purposes. *Generation Zero*, a 2010 documentary produced by the conservative action group Citizens United, blamed the 2008 stock market crash on a baby boomer culture of liberalism, indulgence, and irresponsibility. And a 2010 campaign ad for California Republican gubernatorial candidate Meg Whitman tried to link 1960s antiwar protest imagery to her older Democratic opponent, Jerry Brown.[101]

Liberal boomer critics sometimes scorn their own generation as sell-outs who abandoned youthful idealism and progressive promises for individual gain and greed. Here is sixty-one-year-old liberal comedian Lewis Black: "'The legacy of my generation right now . . . is that we basically have screwed everything up and I don't want to be known as that generation. . . . We made greed kind of acceptable. We destroyed the word 'common good.' We forgot what the social contract is. It's unbelievable. We tore it up. And we were the people who said we were going to make it better. A-ha-ha-ha.'"[102]

Less politically orthodox boomers have also chimed into this critical chorus. The *Washington Post* columnist Robert Samuelson repeatedly chastises his generation for a "policy of selfish silence" on Social Security and Medicare reform.[103] The columnist Joe Queenan skewered fellow baby boomers in his book *Balsamic Dreams*.[104] In (baby boomer) Christopher Buckley's darkly humorous novel *Boomsday*, government-sponsored suicide incentives are suggested as the solution to Social Security's problems.[105]

Members of Generation X joined boomers' self-critique. "Why Don't You All F-Fade Away?" grumbled *Los Angeles Times* editorial writer Meghan Daum. "Even a lot of boomers hate boomers, and not just the right-wing kind, who love to blame the half-life of hippie-era hedonism for everything from teen sex to homelessness." Daum resented being force-fed sixties and seventies pop culture by a "powerful and privileged generation" that considered itself forever young. Her Gen X peers have endured their own realities and problems, such as high levels of student debt and an expensive housing market. As for the incessant 1968 retrospectives, Daum likened them to "an infomercial that endlessly wails, *But wait, there's more!*" Indeed, the fixation upon the 1960s epitomized "the original sin of the baby boom generation: not knowing when to quit."[106] (Another Gen Xer hoped that an Obama-driven political revolution might also displace boomer power in the workplace. "Because once we talk about boomers giving up control of politics, the talk of boomers giving up control of corporate life cannot be far behind.")[107]

As for aging boomers "not knowing when to quit," *Washington Post* columnist Joel Achenbach jokingly called boomers "frisky geezers" following the 2007 arrest of U.S. Senator Larry Craig (age sixty-two) for allegedly making sexual advances to an undercover police officer in a Minneapolis airport restroom. "There are no old people any more," observed Achenbach sarcastically. "Whatever happened to slowing down, sagging into a favorite chair, . . . woodworking in the basement, patrolling the lawn for crab grass?"[108] In the spring of 2009, several high-profile boomer commencement speakers took it upon themselves to issue a generational mea culpa for mismanaging the economy. Speaking at Iowa's Grinnell College, the *New York Times* columnist Thomas Friedman likened his generation to "the grasshopper generation, eating through just about everything like hungry locusts." A contrite Indiana governor Mitch Daniels told Butler University graduates that "all our lives, it's been all about us. . . . We borrowed and splurged and will leave you a staggering pile of bills to pay. . . . It's clear there is no chance that anyone will ever refer to us, as histories now do our parents, as 'The Greatest Generation.'" Even Colorado senator Michael Bennet (barely a boomer by one year at age forty-four), apologized for boomers' greed and irresponsibility. "We lived beyond our means and we are paying a heavy price for that today. . . . We have limited the potential of future generations by burdening them with our poor choices, and our unwillingness to make tough ones."[109]

Along with confessions of generational guilt have come calls for atonement. *New York Times* columnist Nicholas Kristof suggested that boomers might become "Geezers Doing Good," emulating the Microsoft chieftain-turned-philanthropist Bill Gates and devoting the same intensity to a "give-back revolution" that they once did to the sexual revolution.[110] And in an October 2010 *Atlantic* cover story titled "It's the Least We Can Do" Michael Kinsley proposed penance for a profligate generation in the form of a widespread, progressive inheritance tax that would reduce future generations' national debt burden. (His arguments were expanded on the magazine's Web-based forum "on the legacy of boomers and what they owe the country." Most forum participants were boomers critical of boomers.)[111]

What is most significant is that there were few attempts to reject or rebut such public displays of generational guilt. The commencement speeches received some notice—but little else. (The one major exception came from a libertarian who extolled boomers' economic achievements. "This Boomer Isn't Going to Apologize," thundered the economist Stephen Moore on the opinion page of the *Wall Street Journal*.)[112]

There are some indications that this repetitive, negative labeling of aging boomers as "selfish" or "irresponsible" has already taken a toll with the general public. When a Zogby Interactive poll of 4,811 adults were given three choices to define baby boomers' collective legacy, 42 percent chose "ushering in an era of consumerism and self-indulgence," 27 percent chose "helping to bring lasting chance in social and cultural values and ending a war," and the remaining 32 percent were split between the third alternative "nothing at all, nothing really special" and a residual category of "not sure."[113]

This negative generational self-branding is another barrier to positive collective identification and political action. In a sense, aging boomers risk at least partly disarming themselves as a political force in coming battles over entitlement reforms—and the subsequent implementation of those likely changes. Indeed, negative self-labeling as irresponsible and "undeserving" entitlement recipients increases both the certainty and the depth of program cutbacks. Sadly, the well-educated, upper-middle-class propagators of this generational self-deprecation will more easily weather likely age discrimination and Social Security and Medicare cutbacks than their frequent targets—middle- and working-class aging boomers (such as the "Anxious" and "Strugglers" subgroups described in chapter 1).

Boomer Stereotypes by Race and Class

As discussed in the previous chapter, the triumph of Barack Obama highlighted a growing cultural, economic, and political divide. Highly educated, internationally oriented upper-middle-class boomers were smitten with the Obama presidential campaign; large segments of white, small-town, middle- and working-class citizens were not. Both groups were largely, if not predominantly, aging baby boomers. They did not regard one another kindly. To some extent, generational and class stereotypes overlapped.

As mentioned previously, Bill and Hillary Clinton are often seen as the boomer archetype of a highly educated, self-centered ambitious upper middle class. Ivy League–educated Barack Obama, too, was portrayed as an "elitist" or (because of his mixed-race ancestry) as "foreign" or "the other." (Months after his election, disaffected groups continued challenging the authenticity of his birth certificate.) Conversely, mainstream media commentators and pundits ridiculed views and candidates seen as symbolizing small-town or "main street" middle- and working-class Americans. (Presidential candidate Obama was tape-recorded at a San Francisco fund-raiser explaining that the opposition of white, working-class and small-town voters to his candidacy was a frustration-aggression response to economic dislocations. "And it's not surprising, then, they get bitter, they cling to guns or religion or antipathy to people who aren't like them or anti-immigrant sentiment or anti-trade sentiment as a way to explain their frustrations.")[114]

Republican vice presidential candidate Sarah Palin became a lightning rod for channeling heavyweight pundits' contempt for small-town, middle-aged (and older) whites. And the elites loathed the Tea Party movement. The popular *New York Times* columnist Frank Rich took frequent aim at Palin and what she had termed her small-town "real American" base: "Palin stands for a genuine movement: a dwindling white nonurban America that is aflame with grievances and awash in self-pity as the country hurtles into the 21st century and leaves it behind. . . . That resentment is in part about race, of course."[115] Rich's equally popular *New York Times* peer Maureen Dowd constantly savaged Sarah Palin, though Dowd grudgingly acknowledged that the former Alaska governor was good at returning fire, with "a visceral talent for aerial-shooting her favorite human prey: cerebral Ivy League Democrats."[116] (*Washington Post* columnist Richard Cohen compared Palin to the 1950s red-baiter Senator Joseph McCarthy.)[117] Other liberal mainstream commentators' targets included radio talk-show hosts, especially Rush Limbaugh, and personalities at the Fox News Network. (A postelection *Newsweek* magazine cover story featured Limbaugh with his mouth taped shut.)

The stereotype of the small-town or working-class, intolerant, nativist, reactionary who cannot adjust to economic and demographic change is typically an individual or group over age forty or fifty: boomers. That their jobs, career paths, and other economic interests might be genuinely threatened by outsourcing and inexpensive immigrant labor has almost always been ignored or jeered. Along with a disproportionate number of women and minority boomers, members of the white working and middle classes, especially in the deindustrialized Midwest, are the groups most likely to be unprepared for retirement. They will bear the brunt of Medicare or Social Security reductions if these negative class stereotypes morph into "undeserving recipients."

Other boomer subgroups likely to elicit little sympathy are divorced or childless boomers. The demographer Phillip Longman has predicted that large numbers of childless and divorced boomers will constitute "a hidden mass of socially isolated seniors." Younger Americans in an increasingly conservative, religious, and multiethnic America "will tend to view childless Boomers through their parents' eyes; as members of an irresponsible alien tribe. . . . A Boomer without a family will be taken for an aging yuppie, a decaying narcissist, or ailing atheist—none of which stereotypes will be helpful in drawing public sympathy."[118] Longman also warned readers of the looming age/class/ethnic divide emphasized throughout this book: "So on top of the generational divide, on top of the cultural divide, will be a widening racial and ethnic divide."[119]

AND YET: GOOD VIBRATIONS
BETWEEN GENERATIONS

Despite the avalanche of negative stereotyping and bad press, a 2008 Harris Interactive Survey found that Americans' perceptions of baby boomers and older Americans remain surprisingly favorable. Contrary to the media portraits of boomers as self-indulgent and greedy, baby boomers were seen as the generation that was most socially conscious, productive, and "having a positive effect on society." Generation Y (aged thirteen to thirty-one) were thought to be the "most self indulgent" by 53 percent of respondents, followed by Generation X (aged thirty-two to forty-three) at 25 percent; only 18 percent thought boomers were the most self-indulgent.

Thirty-three percent of Harris Interactive respondents felt that the Silent Generation (aged sixty-three to eighty-three) was most admired, followed by the Greatest Generation (over age eighty-four) at 30 percent. The Silent Generation was regarded as the "most generous" by 40 percent, and 33 percent so regarded the baby boomers. Generation X was perceived as the most innovative (41 percent), followed by the baby boomers at 25 percent and Generation Y at 22 percent.

Significantly, more baby boomers (27 percent) were satisfied with their "boomer" title than those in other generational categories. On the other hand, if they could, 40 percent of the Silent Generation would rename themselves the "Responsible Generation."[120]

More important, there is little evidence of serious generational frictions so far. On the contrary, Americans are far more tolerant of generational differences than they once were, especially when compared to the more tumultuous 1960s. Nearly 80 percent of those surveyed in a Pew Research Center study thought there were generational differences. Seventy-three percent thought that young and older people were "very different" in their use of computers and new technology; 69 percent perceived that young and old had "very different" preferences in music; the corresponding figure for "work ethic" was 58 percent, for moral values was 54 percent, and for "respect for others" was 53 percent; the feature on which the least difference was claimed was attitudes toward race and ethnic groups. But these differences were viewed without acrimony. In terms of group frictions, "when compared with other major social divisions, the generation gap ranks at the bottom of the list." Indeed, boomer-era rock and roll music is a common denominator. Though nearly 70 percent saw old and young musical tastes as "very different," nearly two-thirds of all respondents listened to rock and roll—more than any other musical genre.[121] (Another Pew survey published a month later also found low levels of generational tension: only about a quarter of respondents in all age groups felt that conflict between young and old was "very strong" or "strong"; by contrast, an average of 54 percent of all age groups felt that conflict between immigrants and native born was "very strong" or "strong," and an average of 46 percent felt similarly about conflict between rich and poor.)[122]

Existing good vibrations between the generations most assuredly will be tested in the coming years of intensifying entitlement politics.

Aging boomers are entering an increasingly vulnerable period of their lives. Thus far, they are relatively unorganized and unprepared to defend age-based interests. But some individual or organization must do so.

Until and unless aging boomers get their act together, AARP stands ready to be their advocate, arbiter, and supplemental insurance provider—whether boomers like it or not.

CHAPTER FIVE

Not Your Father's AARP

Bill Novelli Builds a New Boomer Brand

> Here's the deal: If you're over 50, for just $12.50 a year, AARP
> will give you a magazine and newsletter subscription, as well
> as allow you to "receive discounts on car rentals, lodging
> cruises" and a host of other wonderful things. And the same
> time, it will argue for your most vital political interests in
> Washington. You're a Republican? Democrat? Anarchist? It
> doesn't matter; it knows what you want. At AARP, one lobby
> fits all.
>
> —Dale Van Atta (2006)

Though the former New York advertising guru Bill Novelli would ini-
tiate substantial organizational and cultural change when he became
AARP's CEO in 2001, Novelli and other AARP spokespersons have
always made sure to regularly, ritually invoke the fifty-year-old organizational mantra "What we do, we do for all." The slogan was established in 1958 by the organization's founder, a former California school
principal, Ethel Percy Andrus (1884–1967), who was outraged by elderly
Americans' poor living conditions and lack of health insurance. Major
speeches by AARP leaders usually contain at least one reverential reference to Andrus, a ritual especially obvious during 2008, when the
organization celebrated its fiftieth year. Despite its enormous growth
in membership, complexity, and political clout, AARP remains rhe-
torically faithful to Andrus's simple, high-minded mission: building

an unusual, hybrid profit/nonprofit "social entrepreneur" organization that sells reasonably priced financial and insurance products to older Americans and then plows the proceeds back into social services, policy advocacy, and an overall "positive aging agenda."

AARP's increasing media presence, its 2005 high-profile campaign against President George W. Bush's Social Security "privatization" reforms, its aggressive boomer and diversity outreach projects, and its very expensive but ultimately successful "Divided We Fail" campaign for comprehensive health care reform are viewed by AARP faithful as well within the context of the historical "big picture." For these loyalists, AARP is still on the course Andrus charted fifty years ago. New CEOs come and go, but Andrus remains a revered, pioneering titan of change who fought the early, decisive battles to found a unique organization and to instill an enduring public service spirit.

Nevertheless, even Andrus probably didn't foresee that AARP would evolve into the nation's second-largest membership organization at forty million (only the Catholic Church is larger)—though critics claim that actual membership may be closer to half of the claimed forty million because dues-paying members' spouses and domestic partners are automatically enrolled. There is little doubt about AARP's lobbying clout: it has been the fourth-highest-spending lobbying group from 1998 to 2009 (ranked second or third highest in four out of six years from 2003 to 2008).[1] It's a remarkable saga.

In 1947, nearly twenty years before the advent of Medicare, Andrus founded the National Retired Teachers Association (NRTA). The original modest mission was to organize a pool of consumers who, collectively, could obtain reasonably priced health insurance. Many retired teachers were too old, sick, or poor to purchase individual policies—some were so impoverished that Andrus allegedly discovered one of them living in a converted chicken coop. Ten years later, NRTA became a subunit in a larger organization offering insurance and a slowly widening range of products to all Americans over fifty: the American Association of Retired Persons (AARP). By 1999, nearly half of all members were still working—so the organization dropped its full name and retained the well-known initials.

In subsequent decades, AARP's fusion of profitable insurance and financial products with social services and policy advocacy has stoked the ire of conservatives bent on curbing or replacing Social Security and Medicare. Following the 1994 "Republican Revolution" electoral landslide, GOP politicians took vengeance via a series of investigations about AARP's conducting for-profit business under its "nonprofit" 501(c)(4) legal status. The former U.S. senator Alan Simpson (R-WY) was especially combative. He grilled AARP officials about the organization's finances and its tax-exempt status. Simpson kept up his criticisms even after retiring from the Senate. "AARP could be such a force for good . . . but they're not. They're selfish, greedy. They don't care about their grandchildren a whit. . . . Now I have the freedom to just beat the brains out of the AARP and I do that all over America."[2]

Simpson's and others' investigations had consequences. In 1994, AARP paid IRS $135 million to settle a dispute over its business income from 1985 through 1993; another $15 million in 1994–95; and still another $52 million in 1999. Also in 1999, the U.S. Postal Service fined AARP for $5.6 million for illegally using nonprofit mailing rates for insurance and other service mailings.[3]

As a result of the 1990s investigations and fines, the main, nonprofit AARP formed two "affiliated entities," the philanthropic AARP Foundation and a for-profit AARP Services. The latter controls licensing and endorsement deals, AARP discounts, and—most important—various forms of health insurance, including its Medicare "Medigap" supplemental policy—in alliance with United Health Services, the largest in the land. In 2006, a new subunit was formed, AARP Financial Services. (AARP's new Global Network also files separate accounting reports.) Membership services remain housed in the nonprofit "mothership," including an increasingly active AARP Grassroots America, the advocacy arm that (quite effectively) mobilizes members who register to receive its e-mails and bulletins. (There is also a "Government Watch" portal that tracks congressional legislation.)

"AARP is powerful because of their sheer numbers," messaging consultant Rich Tau told me. "All they have to do is whisper." The former head of the now defunct Third Millennium association for younger Americans explained, "Even if they mobilize 1 percent of their base, it generates impact and looks very impressive."[4] (Indeed, in its 2009 annual report, AARP proudly states that 1.1 million of its members signed petitions to Congress.)[5]

Tau thinks that AARP is so large that the organization can quickly absorb major policy blunders and simply keep on rolling. (Under Novelli's predecessor, Horace Deets, AARP made two infamous political miscalculations: supporting the ill-fated 1993 Clinton health care reforms and sponsoring the successful enactment of the Medicare Catastrophic Coverage Act in 1988. The latter—intended to provide universal "Medigap" coverage to supplement private policies that varied enormously in terms of adequacy—was hurriedly repealed a year later by Congress after widespread and intensely negative feedback from high-income senior citizens who were hit with substantial Medicare premium increases.)[6] Finally, Tau emphasized: "AARP has no competitors. Conservatives and young people are not predisposed to mobilize collectively."[7]

Conservative activists such as the direct-mail guru Richard Viguerie have tried to establish rival senior organizations: United Seniors Association (now USANext), the Seniors Coalition, and the Sixty-Plus Association. Two newer, conservative AARP alternatives arose during the health care reform battles: the American Seniors Association, headquartered in Atlanta, and the Austin-based Generation America. However, these associations have remained relatively small and ineffective; some appear to be only sporadically active and some have dated Web pages.

The *Wall Street Journal*, the Cato Institute, the Heritage Foundation, the Business Roundtable, and the Concord Coalition have been persistent, sharp AARP critics. "Jabba the AARP," jeered the editorial page of the *Wall Street Journal*, comparing the "great and grabby" organization to the criminal empire of an especially corpulent "Star Wars" villain.[8] In vain.

"Since 1995," Alan Simpson reluctantly concedes, "AARP has gotten stronger, more savvy, more staffed, more alert to their image, hiring more people to soap-suds the American people and their own membership to show that they're doing more and more for the seniors."[9] Simpson credits AARP's continuing success to the work of Bill Novelli, a former New York advertising executive who became AARP's CEO in 2001. Under Novelli, AARP's membership dues increased by 52 percent; its royalties from alliances with insurance and other commercial organizations increased 515 percent. "He [Novelli] is the Wizard of Oz," Simpson admits, and "AARP is a gargantuan marketing organization, a money-making giant."[10]

THE WIZARD OF AARP

The man who transformed AARP for the twenty-first century is Bill Novelli, who, at age sixty, became the CEO in 2001. The co-founder of the famous Porter-Novelli public relations and advertising agency, Novelli brought to AARP a remarkable blend of private- and public-sector leadership experience. He succeeded Horace Deets, a soft-spoken former Catholic priest who guided AARP through twenty years of growth and increasing political confrontation with Republicans and other critics. Changes were already under way to make AARP "Boomer Central" before Novelli arrived. But he considerably expanded and deepened those transformations. Novelli stepped down in 2009, but his impact on organizational restructuring and policy remains very strong.[11]

Novelli's biography is an all-American success story. The son of a steelworker father who once dug graves to support his family during a steel mill strike, Novelli obtained an undergraduate degree from the

University of Pennsylvania and an MA from its Annenberg School for Communications. He began his career working as a salesman for Unilever, then joined a major advertising agency. Eventually, he sought a greater degree of personal fulfillment and social relevance by taking his marketing skills into the public sector—initially as a director of advertising and creative services for the Peace Corps. After a brief foray into political marketing (to reelect Richard Nixon), Novelli and his former Peace Corps boss, Jack Porter, co-founded Porter-Novelli, which quickly become one of the world's largest public relations and advertising agencies. Novelli became known as a marketing "guru" for public service and social causes in both domestic and international realms. He retired from the firm in 1990 and began a second career in the public sector, first as executive vice president of CARE. He next managed the Campaign for Tobacco-Free Kids and then moved to AARP in 2000 as associate executive director of public affairs.[12]

Starting in 2002, Novelli restructured AARP's Washington workforce and began appointing a new executive team and board of directors congruent with helping him achieve three new organizational goals: (1) to be the most successful and acknowledged organization in America for positive social change; (2) to deliver on its promise to each member: to help them make their own choices, reach their goals and dreams, and make the most of life after fifty; and (3) to be a leader in global aging.

Novelli recruited a highly talented and professionalized board of directors, leaders, and staff. Like Novelli, many in this leadership cadre brought a mix of experience in both the private and public sectors in fields ranging from business to health care, government, and social and civic activism. Most board members had had long-term involvement with AARP—some for over twenty years—before ascending to their current position. Nearly every member of the board of directors had achieved distinction at the state or regional level rather than nationally. Several were president of their state AARP. By 2007, one-third of the twenty-four board members were female, and one-third were black, Hispanic, or Asian American.[13]

Novelli closely aligned AARP's agenda with the corporate and political elites' commitments to globalization and internationalism— and also with their deepening concerns about economic polarization and demographic change. Shortly after his appointment as AARP's CEO, Novelli stated that "by serving our members, we serve all generations and, because of the demographic and economic shifts taking place in America and throughout the world, they are more important now than ever before."[14] (Novelli later admitted to me that there was substantial initial resistance to his international emphases from the board of directors.)[15]

Novelli continued Horace Deets's bipartisan outreach, specifically with the former House Republican majority leader, Newt Gingrich. Gingrich nominated Deets to a congressionally appointed commission to recommend changes in Social Security. Deets invited Gingrich to be a featured speaker at AARP's 2002 "Life @ 50+" megaconference in San Diego. Novelli wrote the preface for Gingrich's 2003 health care book, *Saving Lives and Saving Money.* Gingrich was a member of Novelli's advisory bipartisan "kitchen cabinet" that suggested changes at AARP.[16] ("Newt has a new idea every two minutes!" Novelli told me.)

Some left-wing critics suspected that AARP's increasing policy emphases upon markets, technology, and individual control and choice reflected creeping business-Republican bias via the Gingrich-Novelli relationship. When I asked Novelli directly in 2007 about Gingrich's influence, Novelli portrayed himself as a pragmatist interested in "what works" compared to a far more ideologically oriented Gingrich somewhat inflexibly committed to free-market/small-government principles. "What we need is a real dash of cold-water pragmatism," Novelli emphatically told me. "We need a problem-solving perspective instead of [strictly adhering] to the principle that government is good or bad."[17] Novelli channeled his eclectic, can-do pragmatism into two change manifestos designed not only for AARP but for the entire nation.

NOVELLI'S BOOMER REBRANDING CAMPAIGN

As part of Novelli's organizational overhaul and "rebranding" efforts, in 2001 AARP acquired newly crafted vision and mission statements. AARP envisions "a society in which everyone ages with dignity and purpose and in which AARP helps people fulfill their goals and dreams." It is "dedicated to enhancing the quality of life for all as we age. We lead social change and deliver value to members through information, advocacy and service." AARP will help "people 50+ have independence, choice and control in ways that are beneficial and affordable to them and to society as a whole." The organization's revised logo sports an activist, boomer-oriented, social movements theme—"AARP: The power to make it better."[18]

In an era of declining faith in institutions, the public's high level of trust in the AARP brand and reputation is seen by its leaders as paramount; but there is tension between this consumer services brand and a more aggressive "warrior brand," wielded by the organization when it moves more actively into the political and policy arenas.[19]

And Novelli's political and policy agenda for AARP was bold, broad, and ambitious. The two major goals have been transforming the U.S. health care system and helping members achieve long-term financial security. Related to this are helping family caregivers (including adult children caring for older parents and more grandparents taking on child-raising tasks); tackling issues of nursing homes and long-term care; developing "livable communities" amenable to senior citizen needs; addressing ethnic diversity; and encouraging volunteer activities and philanthropy. Defense of Social Security remains steadfast, though the door has been opened to limited changes to preserve the system. And achieving comprehensive health care reform is viewed as an essential first step in preserving Medicare.

AARP's policy agenda has been harnessed to its renowned research and marketing engine, with a direct-mail operation so finely tuned that it locates nearly every American who turns fifty and extends a membership invitation—a darkly humorous rite of passage routinely mocked by late-night television comedians. But it's a good deal. For a mere sixteen-dollar annual membership, AARP offers an expanding bounty of benefits: travel and business discounts, insurance, investment services, low-cost mutual funds, tax assistance, advocacy, civic involvement opportunities, newsletters, and monthly magazines. About seven million people have AARP-branded health insurance, the vast majority being subscribers to Medigap and/or Medicare Part D prescription drug coverage.

By the end of 2009, AARP's total operating revenue was more than $1.4 billion—a nice recovery from $1.08 billion in 2008 due to the stock market decline and an increase from the precrash 2007 total operating revenue of $1.2 billion. About 40 percent of these funds come from royalties and service provider relationship fees with commercial partners—such as United Health Insurance and Metropolitan Life Insurance. The AARP-United Healthcare supplemental insurance for Medicare "Medigap" coverage dominates that market. AARP monitors other organizations that compete with them in terms of both service and advocacy.[20]

AARP's economic and political clout is symbolized by its massive Washington, D.C., headquarters: a block-long, twin-tower, ten-story, Romanesque office structure. Built in 1991 at a cost of $131 million, with more than 820,000 square feet and a high-ceilinged marble lobby, the building houses approximately two thousand employees. So much mail comes and goes that the building has its own zip code. (Once there was spare office space to rent out; no more. AARP's expanding Financial Services Division has spilled over into adjacent buildings.) AARP has offices in every state and citizen chapters in hundreds of locales.

The revamped monthly *AARP Magazine,* which has the largest circulation base in the nation (23.7 million), is a major profit center—in stark contrast to the financial difficulties and bankruptcies confronted daily by other national magazines and publishers. The online version of *AARP Magazine* won a 2009 National Magazine Award for its interactive feature "1968: The Year That Rocked the World." AARP's monthly, issues-oriented *AARP Bulletin* is a newspaper-style publication with a circulation of 24.2 million.[21]

AARP sponsors concerts by famous musicians and advertises on commercial television and PBS programs (such as the nightly *News Hour*). The organization also houses its own profitable media center and produces its own radio and television programs. Most are available on its increasingly sophisticated, information-rich Web page. In 2010, AARP hired former NBC *Today* show host Jane Pauley to anchor a monthly television segment, "Your Life Calling," and to moderate the new Web site offering AARP.org/Jane. Both the television segment and the Web site focus upon how people are reinventing themselves and "trying new things." *AARP Magazine* sponsors an annual "Movies for Grown-Ups" awards show that has obtained a measure of Hollywood clout.

AARP recently expanded its Latino-oriented, Spanish-language media through AARP VIVA. The new enterprise will expand upon AARP's Spanish-language quarterly magazine *Segunda Juventud* and into radio, the Web, and television, including a new hourlong Spanish-language television series, *Viva su Segunda*. And AARP is going global as its Global Network division is linking up with similar organizations worldwide, including the Canadian Association for Fifty-Plus (CARP), Italy's Fenacom, and Copenhagen-based Daneage. A primary purpose is to share research and information, but AARP for-profit services may also go global. It may become somewhat apt to wryly observe that "the sun never sets on the AARP empire."[22] (However, the empire was not immune to the stock market crash and the Great Recession. In 2009, AARP suffered its worst financial setback in history, which resulted in layoffs of 10 percent of its staff and cutbacks in all major programs.)

AARP aims to have a membership that mirrors the nation's fifty-plus population, but it remains disproportionately middle class and about 88 percent white. Nearly half the members are under age sixty-five; the average age of all members is sixty-four; and they join AARP at an average age of fifty-four. About 32 percent have at least "some college" and another 33 percent have at least a four-year college degree. Nearly one-third of members work full time, and only 47 percent are retired; half of member households earn $50,000 and 28 percent earn $75,000 or more. Eighty percent own their homes.[23] Inasmuch as men die earlier than women, there is a female tilt to membership, 55 to 45 percent. (Female members seem to be more active participants in the organization, especially in volunteering and in attending AARP "Life @ 50+" annual megaconferences). AARP officials would like to increase the 58 percent renewal rate for first-time members (about average for similar organizations). Attracting Hispanics and blacks remains problematic: in 2008, only 5.6 percent of members were African American, 4.1 percent were Hispanic, and only 1.4 percent were "non-Hispanic Asian."[24]

AARP is increasingly pondering its postboomer future. Its "Future Champions" campaign was launched to raise AARP awareness and allegiance among younger, more ethnically diverse Americans. That is the strategy behind the television advertisements featuring people of all ages and ethnicities who happily inform viewers that "AARP is for everyone who has a birthday." "Project Prepare" was a major new AARP research effort to map the characteristics and needs of the under-fifty population. The same multigenerational mission undergirded the high-budget "Divided We Fail" campaign for comprehensive health care reform (focus group tested, crafted, and launched in alliance with the Business Roundtable and the Service Employees International Union).

The culmination of AARP's research and outreach to younger generations was the 2009 launch of its "Lifetuner" Web page (www .lifetuner.org), designed to encourage younger Americans to become "financially literate" and consider "8 Money Habits for Lifelong Financial Health" (especially in saving for retirement via the new norm of individual retirement accounts). The site gives AARP yet another rebranding tweak designed to deflect its "greedy geezer" stereotype by proclaiming: "Lifetuner is brought to you by AARP, a non-profit dedicated to helping people of all ages make smarter choices today for a better life tomorrow."

Novelli's increasingly busy, multipurpose agenda, coupled with intensified drives for greater ethnic diversity, generational inclusiveness, and international alliances, led some senior-level staff to worry about loss of identity and mission. "Why don't we just re-name ourselves the 'American Association of Persons'?" was a sarcastic, *sotto voce* complaint I occasionally heard.

Overall, though, the board members, management team, and staff members with whom I spoke seemed remarkably happy to be working for AARP—despite what one officer termed "the loss of a family feeling" due to recent reorganization and downsizing. There is limited in-house grumbling about what some perceive as a growing subordination of policy and research functions to the business-services ends of the organization. And some voiced the oft-heard suspicion of outside critics that "AARP is really all about making money." Yet it was the savvy combination of forward-looking policy research and marketing acumen that led AARP to anticipate and assess the boomer age wave and its many consequences—long before any other institution took note.

But will AARP be aging boomers' ally, championing their interests? Or is AARP more likely to broker and compromise boomers' concerns as the organization increasingly eyes the financial needs and future political preferences of a younger, more diverse America?

INSURANCE AGENT OR POLITICAL ADVOCATE?

AARP's fusion of financial products services with politics draws its sharpest conflict-of-interest critics on the political right; but there are those on the political left as well. The *American Prospect* author Barbara Dreyfuss regarded Novelli's ascent with suspicion. She saw Novelli's bipartisanship tilt as part of an ongoing "seduction" of the organization by business and Republicans. She found that Novelli had "centralized policy making by limiting input from local AARP leaders and brought with him a team of corporate executives to run the group's federal and state policy—people much more comfortable with Republicans, open to private plans and market-oriented policies and more willing to make deals than many of the veteran staff."[25] Dreyfuss was especially galled by the Novelli and Newt Gingrich association.

Dreyfuss's article reflected liberal anger and betrayal over Novelli's controversial decision in 2003 to throw AARP's support behind a Republican-driven, business-friendly Medicare Prescription Drug and Modernization Act. The act created new Medicare prescription drug coverage plans largely administered by private insurers—the largest of which would turn out to be AARP's own brand of Medicare supplementary insurance (in partnership with United Health). The legislation provided good coverage to those with low or high levels of pharmaceutical needs but permitted a sizable coverage gap (the so-called "donut hole") for those with moderate-to-heavy needs. The act also prohibited bargaining for low drug prices between Medicare and pharmaceutical companies and authorized more widespread offerings of insurance featuring individually managed health savings accounts.

Novelli and AARP's officers defended their actions on the organization's Web page, in AARP magazines, and at the Life @ 50+ conferences. Their rationale was that the Medicare Modernization Act was the best deal they could obtain at the time—that half a loaf was better than none. Novelli and his team were well aware that Bush wanted to tout this accomplishment in his reelection campaign; and they also knew that if Medicare reforms weren't enacted in 2003, and if Bush won reelection in 2004, there would likely be no reform at all. Nevertheless, sixty thousand AARP members reportedly resigned in protest, and Beltway liberals fumed that AARP had caved in to a conservative agenda of privatizing Medicare and gutting employer-provided health insurance.[26]

In 2005 Novelli steered AARP back toward its New Deal ideological moorings, vigorously defending traditional Social Security against President George W. Bush's efforts to open the program to privately managed equity accounts. As opposed to AARP's hesitant "neutrality" on proposed Social Security reforms during the 1990s, Novelli's campaign featured a devastating television advertisement featuring a woman who summons a plumber to fix a clogged sink—only to have her entire house demolished. (The obvious message was that Social Security has minor problems requiring a limited fix, not total destruction.) This successful campaign partially mollified disgruntled liberals inside and outside AARP—and, once more, infuriated conservatives.[27]

In late 2008, however, AARP again aroused critics' "money machine" suspicions when it became the target of a lawsuit and an investigation by Senator Charles Grassley (R-IA), who was responding to constituent complaints about AARP/United Healthcare limited-benefit and indemnity health insurance policies. Sold under the names of Medical Advantage, Essential Plus, and Hospital Indemnity Plan, the policies were designed as essentially supplemental coverage for early retirees in their fifties and early sixties. People who bought the policies charged that the limited nature of the policies wasn't made clear.

Grassley and his staff conducted an investigation of AARP using "secret shoppers." He concluded that "AARP is systematically misleading its members by failing to ensure that they are fully apprised of the risks and underinsurance associated with indemnity plans that are being sold under its name."[28] In January 2009, Bloomberg News aired a critical, hourlong expose based on the lawsuit and Grassley's investigations titled "AARP: Making Money, Losing Trust."

Fortunately for AARP, the controversy faded rather quickly. And the Bloomberg expose was balanced by a largely positive CBS Moneywatch four-part series on AARP's mutual funds, life insurance and annuities, auto and homeowners' insurance, and health and long-term care insurance.[29]

But the Bloomberg "Losing Trust" documentary title stung. Trust is the paramount value for AARP's "member value" division—and its legal staff. And they are not necessarily pleased when AARP's leaders take the organization into battles in controversial policy terrain.

BATTLE OF THE BRANDS: CONSUMER TRUST
VERSUS POLICY WARRIOR

AARP's dual business/politics model leads not only to conflict-of-interest charges but also to competing organizational identities—or "brands," in the lingo of Novelli's public relations field. These dual personalities continue to make AARP "a seriously schizoid organization"—a diagnosis made more than a dozen years ago by Charles Morris.[30] To maximize its consumer base, AARP's products-and-services "member value" function requires high levels of nonpartisan public trust unsullied by controversy. But strong political stands or controversial compromises required for political advocacy—what Novelli terms the "warrior brand"—jeopardize broad public trust and risk alienating politically attuned customers.

Midway through Novelli's tenure as CEO, AARP was still struggling to integrate these competing "member value" and "social impact" agendas—a tension quite evident in the organization's 2006 "Strategic Plan."[31] This organizational blueprint blends a general social change outlook with a more market- and choice-oriented, risk-shift America. Thus, in addition to being a "champion brand to enrich the lives of all people and enhance society as a whole," AARP is also a partner that "helps people navigate life's on-going and changing needs (health, finances, connecting, giving, enjoying)."

"Engagement on social issues" is one the five major goals of member value. The latter has its own set of four goals: (1) economic security—ensuring a Social Security that is solvent for the long term, enabling age fifty-plus Americans to remain in the workforce, helping Americans accumulate and manage retirement assets, and protecting low-income and vulnerable populations; (2) health and supportive services—promoting quality health care access and coverage and encouraging improved health status through healthy behaviors; (3) livable communities—encouraging local governments and business to provide affordable and appropriate housing options and to sustain mobility options for aging populations for whom driving is problematic; and (4) global aging—encouraging governments to better serve the needs of older citizens and informing businesses of the needs, talents, interests, and marketing possibilities of older populations.

Insofar as the social impact and member value agendas overlap on providing information and services, a nonpartisan, noncontroversial brand works fine. But the social impact goals of maintaining economic security (including Social Security) and quality health care for age fifty-plus Americans (through general health care reform and through Medicare) are inextricably linked to AARP's policy advocacy and its "warrior brand."

AARP's legal and media relations departments are hawkish in protecting the nonpartisan consumer trust brand. The two departments seem extremely cautious and conservative. Not only are they understandably sensitive about public relations gaffes, but they have reasonable fears of "deep pockets" lawyers looking for excuses to sue the forty-million-member organization. Thus AARP's legal department has reportedly come to exercise an extraordinary amount of control over routine communications of AARP staff with outsiders, even by AARP's resident scholars and researchers. (The only two AARP officials who refused to be interviewed for this book first sought official permission through "legal.")[32]

AARP's legal and media relations departments are also wary of long-term foes such as the former U.S. senator Alan Simpson (R-WY), who loves to tweak the tensions between AARP's business and policy advocacy goals. Simpson is fond of deflating AARP's claim that it represents the political interests of its millions of members with his trademark jeer that AARP's members are merely "bound together by a common love of airline discounts and automobile discounts and RV discounts."[33]

At least one AARP board member ruefully acknowledged a good measure of truth in Simpson's putdown. But the former senator's characterization has also served as a call to action. AARP leaders not only want boomers' membership fees and business; they also covet boomers' political respect and, especially, boomers' *trust*. This is why, more than a decade ago, AARP officials set out to make AARP "Boomer Central."[34]

TRANSFORMING THE BOOMERS:
FROM "ME" TO "WE"

For the past decade, and probably throughout the next one, AARP's most vital task is to recruit and retain aging baby boomers. Attracting and keeping members of this keenly consumer-oriented and politically volatile generation is vital to AARP's survival. There is an understandably high mortality rate when members must be at least fifty years old to join: two million die each year. Therefore, the organization has a special imperative to "grow or perish." Since 2000, AARP has more than compensated by adding more than 2.5 million new members annually via its famously thorough direct-mail campaigns—increasingly supplemented by television advertisements and a sophisticated Web page.

The key task for AARP has been to transform middle-aged boomers' competitive individualism and relative lack of interest in civic involvement into social activism and the desire to "leave a legacy" through working with others. AARP's leaders believe that, as boomers enter retirement and old age, there might be a partial revival of the 1960s' change heritage. Chief operating officer Tom Nelson insisted to me that "boomers want to be a part of something that has impact." An oft-heard slogan was "Changing 'me' into 'we.'"

Even before Novelli's appointment as CEO in 2001, an organizational facelift called "Today's AARP" was under way to attract baby boomers. First to go was the dowdy *Modern Maturity* magazine that boomers grimly remember seeing on their parents' coffee tables. For about two years new boomer members received a separate, slick monthly publication entitled *My Generation*. The response, however, was underwhelming. *My Generation* disappeared and boomer members were integrated into the mailing list for a retitled and substantially revised general monthly publication *AARP: The Magazine*—quietly tailored to different age subgroups in terms of format, style, and content. A Spanish-language monthly magazine, *Segunda Juventad,* was also launched—recently complemented by a Spanish-language television broadcast. As mentioned above, all of AARP's publications and radio and television programs are available online at AARP.org, a repeatedly upgraded and increasingly sophisticated Web site. The result: one-third of AARP is now under age sixty.

Though AARP is a huge organization, its drive since 2000 to become "Boomer Central" was originally initiated by one man: AARP's director of strategy and public policy, John Rother, a savvy and tireless Capitol Hill veteran and political tactician.

AARP'S Boomer Brain

"Most Americans haven't heard of John Rother, but he may have more influence than most senators when it comes to Social Security," observed the *New York Sun* reporter Luiza Savage. AARP's sixty-four-year-old executive vice president of policy, strategy, and international affairs is a bearded, affable man, the son of a Methodist minister, a graduate of Oberlin College and the University of Pennsylvania Law School.

Rother has become known as a skilled negotiator and a mild-mannered lobbyist who practices the art of "maintaining good lines of communication with everyone"—especially with Congress. He honed such skills by working there. For eight years he was special counsel for labor and health to former senator Jacob Javits. He then became staff director and chief counsel for the Special Committee on Aging under its chairman, Senator John Heinz. He moved to AARP in 1984 and has also become a member of several boards and commissions dealing with aging and health care.

The energetic Rother's wide span of Washington contacts ranges from the president of the United States to Hans Riemer, the former Washington director of "Rock the Vote." Riemer cooperated with

Rother on a massive 2005 public relations campaign to defeat George
W. Bush's efforts to creative private accounts within Social Security.
Reimer characterizes Rother as "inspirational" and as a central figure in the social welfare policy community. (Reimer later joined
the staff of AARP's "Create the Good" Web site that is geared to
promoting volunteerism.)

Rother was the prime mover in getting AARP to anticipate the
advent of the boomer age wave, to understand how that generation was
different from older constituents—and how to appeal to them.[35] Rather
like CEO Bill Novelli, Rother is a somewhat center-left pragmatist who
firmly insists that "politics is the art of the possible."

I interviewed and talked informally with Rother many times over
the past decade. He probably understands his generational peers better than anyone else in the nation. He is adept at grasping underlying common characteristics and outlooks rooted in boomers' shared
childhood and young adult experiences—while trying to avoid over-
generalizations about a huge age cohort subdivided by gender, class,
education, race/ethnicity, and religion. In this effort, he has had the aid
of AARP's large and talented research staff. (AARP has so much more
data about boomers than any other American institution that they have
undertaken a major outreach to corporate America by forming "Focalyst" in partnership with the New York–based research and consulting
Kantar Group.)

According to Rother, boomers did not share a widespread defining experience similar to their parents' widespread hardship of the
Great Depression followed the common cause and sacrifices demanded
during World War II. Instead, raised in postwar prosperity, boomers
became fiercely individualistic, wanting to be in charge and in control of their own lives. "Boomers want options and choices," Rother
explained. "They're optimistic, self-reliant, and self-indulgent."

Rother described boomers' cultural identity as very loose, built primarily around their shared musical heritage. He didn't sense a case for
boomer political activism—yet. But during our first conversation in

late 1999 the prescient policy analyst predicted the likely precipitating crisis: "Health care is going to be the dominant issue of the next decade if not beyond." Boomers would be in the thick of it.

Rother was pleased to point out that boomers had already rebelled against managed care restrictions. "{hrs}'Hard' managed care—with gatekeepers and other restrictions," explained Rother, "goes against the core elements of boomer culture, of 'doing it my way' and making choices. The 1990s HMOs just punched into that—pow!"

Boomers led the attack on hard-line HMOs formats and propelled the trend toward "soft" managed care with higher expenses and deductibles—but more options and patient choice. "And that's what Medicare is!" Rother beamed triumphantly. Boomers will warm to Medicare because "it provide menus, options, discounting, and choice."

Rother the optimist hoped that boomers' inherent distrust of large institutions and especially government might lessen as they learned to access and use Social Security and Medicare. (As seen in the next chapter, in the aftermath of the battle for health care reform and the rise of the Tea Party, Rother would have to reconsider this view.) On the other hand, Rother the realist has always acknowledged that Medicare would have to cut costs and become more efficient and decentralized. Like Bill Novelli and Newt Gingrich, however, Rother had faith in new technologies and increased individual health awareness in reducing high costs. He was more pessimistic about boomer-driven changes in family structure upon an aging America—fewer children, more working women, more divorce, blended families, and geographical dispersion.

"No caregivers," he grimly conceded.

Like nearly all high-level AARP personnel, Rother once told me he found the possibility of generational warfare "far-fetched"—at least insofar as economic conditions remained stable. In subsequent years, however, he mused more darkly that "the system pits groups against each other." Partly for that reason—and Americans' inherent mistrust of government—Rother has always discounted the ability of the United States to adopt a Canadian-style, government-run, universal health insurance system. "I tell liberal friends to get over it." (He would have to restate that rationale repeatedly as AARP ramped up a "Divided We Fail" campaign that totally ignored a Canadian alternative.)

AARP's Office of Social Impact built upon Rother and his "research shop's" inputs to arrive at a general consensus on boomer concerns: boomers and older Americans wish to have the security choices and control to help them live actively, independently, and purposively for as long as they can. They want to leave their children and grandchildren and the nation a better place than when they found it—and not be a burden to anyone. (The office developed a series of measurable benchmark strategy goals to respond to these needs: economic security, health security and supportive services, livable communities, information and resources, and international leadership.)

Twin Manifestos: To Preserve Medicare, Reform Health Care

Though Novelli has labored mightily to make AARP's image more pragmatic, bipartisan, and open to "anyone who has a birthday," big-name pundits continue to attack AARP's "greedy geezer" stereotype. First and foremost is *Washington Post* columnist Robert Samuelson, who regularly charges that AARP is the "nation's most dangerous lobby": "Among AARP's 36 million members, there must be many decent people who benefit from the 5 to 50 percent discounts. . . . But I won't be joining because AARP has become America's most dangerous lobby. If left unchecked, its agenda will plunder our children and grandchildren. Massive outlays for the elderly threaten huge tax increases and other government spending. Both may weaken the economy and the social fabric. No thanks . . . AARP's America is an illusion. Sooner or later it will be overtaken by demographic and economic realities."[36]

AARP's strategy to counter such critical blasts was formulated in two publications. *Reimagining America: How America Can Grow Old and Prosper* (2005) was an in-house report, a "blueprint for the future." One year later, much of it was recast as a heavily publicized, popular-audience book by Novelli titled *50+: Igniting a Revolution to Reinvent America* (2006).[37]

Novelli's book was a relentlessly upbeat and optimistic manifesto, a "call to action" aimed at baby boomers' social movement heritage and appealing to their desire to turn "me into we" and leave a lasting legacy. Novelli also targeted boomers' cultural preferences for individual responsibility, choice, and consumer empowerment. The book's can-do, get-it-done spirit was activated in the book's foreword written by the high-tech entrepreneur and AOL founder Steve Case.

The central purpose in both Novelli's book and *Reimagining America* was to confront and redefine the "overstated" entitlement problem posed by Samuelson and other prophets of doom: "Can America afford to grow old? And can we do so with intergenerational fairness, without burdening our children and grandchildren with the bills?" The answer was "yes"—if appropriate political and individual steps were taken.[38]

The tasks of preserving Medicare and Social Security were portrayed as "opportunities" to transform the health care system, lifestyles, the workplace, and retirement.[39] Social Security could be sustained through relatively minor adjustments; Medicare could be preserved through comprehensive reforms of the entire American health care system by harnessing the curative power of preventive care, encouraging technological innovation, developing "best practices" medical standards, implementing market and consumer-driven changes, and encouraging individual healthy lifestyles. ("To some extent, we can expect the marketplace to resolve these issues. The growing number of older consumers as the baby boomers age will create demands that smart business owners will hasten to answer.")[40]

Both *50+: Igniting a Revolution to Reinvent America* and *Reimagining America* clearly pulled AARP away from its implicit commitment to Franklin Delano Roosevelt's New Deal liberalism, with its faith in big-government solutions to social problems; instead, there was movement back toward Theodore Roosevelt's earlier progressive vision of individual-business-government cooperation and personal action and responsibility.[41]

Indeed, and perhaps most significantly, both *Reimagining America* and Novelli's *50+* did not mention the capstone dream of the New Deal and Great Society heritage: government-funded, universal health care. Instead, proposed reforms aimed to increase access to and affordability of a system modified by large doses of boomer-based faith in markets, individual responsibility and choice, and technology: themes that would be echoed in the massive "Divided We Fail" health care reform campaign—and later the Democrats' health care reform proposals.

Likewise, these two blueprint documents contained little protest about the decline of lifetime, "defined-benefit" pensions by the nation's corporations. Instead, the twin manifestos urged employers to automatically enroll employees in 401(k) individual retirement accounts—rather than putting the initiative on the individual. Employers were also urged to provide more flexible time schedules and phased retirement plans. Employees were encouraged to save more and work longer.

On Social Security reforms, *Reimagining America* moved back to more traditionally liberal options that included (1) raising the percentage of earnings subject to payroll tax to 90 percent; (2) raising the dollar amount of earnings security payroll taxes from $90,000 to $120,000, including a 3 percent surtax over that amount; (3) indexing benefits—reducing benefits for higher-wage workers; and (4) taxing Social Security benefits like private pensions. "Personalizing" Social Security by diverting contributions into private accounts was rejected outright.

Despite the chatter of change, when all was said and done, Bill Novelli's AARP still defended existing Medicare and Social Security programs by invoking the stark alternative: "The question really ought to be how can we afford *not* to sustain the monumental contributions these programs have made to the health and well being of America's aged population?"[42] And tucked away at the end of *Reimagining America* was a return to a New Deal remedy: raising taxes. ("Respected parties across the political spectrum all recognize that the long-term outlook is bleak unless we raise additional revenues.").[43]

AARP'S TRAVELING CIRCUS: THE ANNUAL LIFE @ 50+ EVENTS

AARP's social impact foci and the rest of its evolving, boomer-friendly agenda and image were gradually rolled out, refined, and tested at a series of annual megaconferences titled "Life @ 50+." Beginning in 2001, these conferences ostensibly showcased AARP's vast array of products and services as well as providing forums for its policy advocacy. Behind the scenes, AARP was also doing focus group research on its products, its policy positions, and the conference itself, testing the reception of various celebrities, star keynote speakers, panel topics, and evening big-name entertainment acts. The early conferences provided a window into AARP's delicate balancing act of wooing baby boomers while also maintaining relationships with older members and AARP's many other political and economic clienteles.

The first 2001 Life @ 50+ conference in Dallas was something of a flop, drawing only six thousand people. The 2002 Life @ 50+ conference, however, attracted nearly fourteen thousand paid registrants (at fifteen dollars a ticket) to the giant San Diego Convention Center. Just as importantly, the average age of attendees dropped from seventy-two to sixty-six. There were 272 exhibitors, nearly one hundred more than the year before. In the subsequent years, the three-day events became a major marketing success, drawing larger crowds of twenty-five thousand or more; as aging boomers took a greater interest, the average age declined to a relatively "young" sixty-two.

People were drawn to the conferences for a variety of reasons. "I'm here to meet broads," declared Bill, a divorced, sixty-year-old luncheon companion at the San Diego conference. Bill (a pseudonym) had led a busy life as a father of five and a traveling computer programmer and entrepreneur. Bill claimed that his wife couldn't put up with his travel schedule so they had divorced. He had acquired a girlfriend but had grown weary of her time-consuming, unsuccessful attempt to rehabilitate her drug-addicted son. "I'm not sure I'll get married again," said Bill. "Right now, I just want to find someone to go on cruises with."

The gender ratio at the San Diego event (and most other Life @ 50+ conferences) favored Bill's quest. More than 60 percent were women, as were 90 percent of the two hundred or so people who packed a workshop entitled "Dating after 50" by Tom Blake, newspaper columnist and author of *Fifty and Dating Again*. Blake pointed out the obvious reason for the rising female-to-male ratio among those over fifty: men die sooner. By age sixty-five, he explained, half of women are widows, and they complain that the dwindling number of prospective second husbands want a "nurse and a purse." Nevertheless, Blake urged older women seeking relationships to be optimistic but realistic, get out the house, network, and be positive and "mentally available." He was leery of singles clubs and the Internet. "Don't expect someone to make your life better." Above all, remember that, if all else fails, "being single isn't so bad."

A major feature of the "Life @ 50+" conferences was an annual all-star "2011 Panel" (so-named for the year in which oldest boomers turn sixty-five). The first 2011 panel at San Diego featured the actor/activist Bill Baldwin, the *Washington Post*–famed "Watergate" reporter Carl Bernstein, the *Fear of Flying* feminist novelist Erica Jong, the generations expert William Strauss, and the Brandeis law professor Anita Hill. Mostly, they argued. The panelists displayed little agreement about boomers' key characteristics and attitudes—or anything else. Strauss offered the generalization that boomers reflected America's postwar prosperity's idealism and individualism. Bernstein immediately disagreed, emphasizing that the vast generation was deeply divided between older Vietnam-era boomers and their younger, postwar siblings. Anita Hill questioned whether boomers had enacted deep institutional change and produced effective politicians. Erica Jong contradicted Hill with examples of boomer presidents Bill Clinton and

George W. Bush. Strauss sparked sharp disagreement from other panelists when he cited polling data showing that boomers were becoming more promilitary.

The 2004 Life @ 50+ in Las Vegas was the most star-studded convention yet. It would also attract one of highest registrations of any of the conferences before or after—twenty-seven thousand attendees. The evening entertainment headliners had a distinctly Older Baby Boomers tilt: the Smothers Brothers, Motown original Smokey Robinson, and blues singer James Taylor—the latter hurriedly evacuated from the auditorium at the end of his performance when enthusiastic AARP members rushed the stage. "When I saw that," remembered chief operating officer Tom Nelson, "I turned to a couple of board members sitting near me and said, 'This is a turning point. AARP members are rocking out!'"

The Vegas event was bankrolled by even more major corporate players: Gateway Computers, Pillsbury, and Proctor and Gamble joined prior sponsors Anheuser-Bush, Home Depot (now partners with AARP Foundation in forming a National Hiring Partnership program to employ senior citizens), and United Health Group (AARP's health insurance partner). The television film critic Roger Ebert hosted an "AARP Celebrates Cinema" series. The Hollywood film star Danny Glover would be featured at the exhibit hall presentation "Voices of Civil Rights," a project preserving all manner of records and documents from the American civil rights movement, co-sponsored by AARP, the National Conference on Civil Rights, and the Library of Congress. The veteran comedian Jerry Lewis would host a session called "Making the Most of Life." The "AARP University" series featured sessions on AARP's role in enacting the controversial new Medicare prescription drug plan, a session reflecting AARP's civic involvement push, "Bet on Community Service!" and a panel on sex and aging featuring the television personality Dr. Ruth Westheimer.

Though not on the preconference program, the Democratic presidential nominee John Kerry and First Lady Laura Bush appeared.

(President George Bush was also in Vegas but wisely avoided a potentially chilly reception by sending Laura.) The First Lady proved to be a remarkably poised speaker and was accorded an increasingly warm reception. But Kerry was the obvious favorite, initially greeted by loud ovations that grew progressively less so as he droned on too long—for fifty minutes.

The greatest public relations bomb at any of the Life @ 50+ conferences detonated in Vegas: a tempestuous annual 2011 boomer panel featuring the opinionated Hollywood star Cybill Shepherd.

The *AARP Magazine* editor Hugh Delahanty initially opened the panel by playfully asking, "What will baby boomers do when they grow up?" Steve Gillon, a professor and History TV host and author of the just-published *Boomer Nation,* offered a scholarly description of boomers as a diverse generation, animated by a "culture of choice" and individualism. Though still divided over the 1960s culture wars, boomers were conservative in many ways. He offered the baby boomer Newt Gingrich as an example.

"Newt climbed out of a swamp!" Cybill Shepherd jeered loudly. When the humorist Christopher Buckley mentioned the legacy of Vietnam, Shepherd sharply interrupted again: "We all agree about Vietnam: a *waste!*" Then she added for no apparent reason that women thought differently than men.

Donna Brazile, the shrewd African American strategist who managed Al Gore's presidential campaign, described boomers as becoming more ambivalent about the changes they had set in motion in the 1960s. "They're wondering: Is change good?" She agreed with Gillon that boomers might be turning more conservative but also turning away from politics.

Shepherd contradicted Brazile's contentions about boomer political ambivalence. "Fifty-seven of boomers support choice!" she stated emphatically. "We are *not* divided! Bush wants to repeal choice! We're fed up with it! This president was *not* elected!" As a trickle of walkouts was becoming a stream, Shepherd suddenly shifted to how liberated women regard plastic surgery. "We can wear our breasts up or down," she declared proudly. "It depends on 'How do I feel about myself?'" Christopher Buckley gamely chimed in that "we worry about a shortage of flu vaccine, but the problem may be a botox shortage."

Delahanty shifted the topic onto how "boomers redefine life stages." Gillon emphasized the point of his book *Boomer Nation* that boomers are ambivalent about big government: "We look to Washington, but distrust it—fear it won't provide funds in our old age."

"It gets better as you get older," mused Donna Brazille, soberly reflecting on her birth in New Orleans Charity Hospital to a mother who had nine children—a mother who ultimately died at age fifty-two in the same hospital. Cybill Shepherd had a different view of women's life passages. "Maidens, mothers, crones," she quipped. "At forty," she declared, "things change." This was a segue to closing the panel with a song she'd written, "The Menopause Blues." But not before another blast at George W. Bush. "Spit rolls downhill!" she cried. "I despise this president! He favors the rich! He talks about separation of church and state. Yet he wants to mess with states' rights [on abortion] and my rights as a woman!"

From behind Shepherd, her exasperated fellow panelist Christopher Buckley softly pleaded, "Shut up and sing!"

Shepherd whirled on him. "'Shut up and sing' is an insult! You've offended my sense of womanhood!" She berated him a bit more in this vein.[44] Then the pianist began to play and Shepherd began her rather bawdy ballad, typified by the following lyrics:

> If you're feeling dry,
> Just make yourself a drink!
>   Splash vermouth and estrogen, it's later than you think!
> I've got those menopause blues, those ol' menopause blues!
>   You can keep your Viagra! Testosterone, too!
> My libido's on the rise, there's honey pourin' through!

The pace of audience walkouts quickened. Most of those exiting were white-haired folk who were plainly disgusted. The remaining audience members applauded modestly. Several rushed to the stage, mainly to visit or get autographs from Brazile or Shepherd—the latter appeared to have intimidating bodyguards.

Virtually all AARP officials I interviewed downplayed cultural or political generational tensions within AARP or the broader society. But Shepherd's polarizing performance became the talk of the conference, and AARP officials who attended the 2004 Vegas conference still wince when the episode is recalled.

At the 2006 Life @ 50+ conference in Anaheim (described in the introductory chapter), the 2011 panel was assembled for the final time. The panelists were more sedate and reflective, focusing on boomers' relationship to popular culture.[45] There was some griping about ageism on Madison Avenue and Hollywood. The former Motown executive and now independent producer Suzanne de Passe complained that boomer-oriented films were a very tough sell. On the other hand, Larry W. Jones, president of TV Land and Nick at Night, had happily capitalized upon boomer-era nostalgia television programming. He admitted that such fare was "pure escapism"—but drew a laugh from the audience when he observed that "our ratings go up as the rest of television gets crappier."

Ken Burns, producer of several documentary series for PBS, spoke movingly about boomers searching for continuity and community through music and memory. The music and entertainment of their youth, Burns observed, trigger memories of where they were and whom they were with—parents, family, friends. Shared entertainment and memories link the generations. Burns was surprised at the large numbers of boomers like himself who remained fascinated with their parents' experiences and memories of World War II, the focus of *The War,* his then-current nine-part documentary. And today, he laughed, "if I can get my hands on my kids' iPod, I find they're downloading the Beatles."

So far, Burns mused, the boomers' story was being felt—via memory and nostalgia—more than being actively told or debated. But AARP researchers knew that boomers' story was about to be told more darkly and seriously. It was going to be "felt" through increasing fiscal and physical pain.

"If you could point to a single type of event and cost that is the greatest source of life stage angst, it is a health care crisis and associated costs," AARP's senior vice president for thought leadership Jody Holtzman later told me. "There are two aspects of it. One is the financial issue—even when you assume you're covered. All you need is a big bill or deductible—say $2,000. For the average household, that's a lot of money when it's cash off the top. And, for older boomers, associated with that might be a serious health outcome. That all of a sudden, they realize, 'I can't do what I did before, I can't do it as easily, I can't do it in the same way' . . . can't play basketball or even walk around the block. Then you start playing out the scenario. Once you start playing out the scenario—health problems and cost—you begin to wonder: 'Is this the beginning of a snowball?' Then comes the angst."[46]

TRANSFORMING HEALTH CARE: LAUNCHING "DIVIDED WE FAIL"

In 2007 AARP launched "Divided We Fail," a coalition for health care reform that included the Business Roundtable, the Service Employees International Union, and the National Federation of Independent Businesses. AARP's chief operating officer Tom Nelson explained to me that "we ramped up 'Divided We Fail' to build unexpected coalitions with groups like labor and business and to bridge generational interests and create a powerful movement for health care reform."

As seen in previous chapters, aging baby boomers have become increasingly anxious about health care reform because they are entering the highly vulnerable fifty to sixty-five age range. Individual insurance policies on the open market for someone in that age range are extremely expensive and often impossible to obtain if there are preexisting health conditions. AARP had begun offering (through United Healthcare

Insurance Company) a range of high-deductible policies for those aged fifty to sixty-four.

The overriding problem for the Divided We Fail coalition was: How to sell health care reform to a skeptical public?

How to Talk to the Public about Health Care Reform, an AARP PowerPoint lecture, provided a window into the research and strategy behind the Divided We Fail campaign. The AARP director of policy and strategy, John Rother, AARP board president-elect Jennie Chin Hansen, and board member Joanne Handy presented the talk at the 2007 Chicago Joint Conference of the American Society on Aging/National Conference on Aging.[47]

The AARP presenters first established the case for health care reform, especially for age fifty-plus Americans. A bar chart illustrated that uninsured Americans aged fifty to sixty-four constituted the fastest-growing segment of all forty-seven million uninsured Americans. Successive charts and graphs starkly portrayed current and growing inadequacies in the American health care system: (1) boomers' health care costs would increase as they aged, while their incomes would decline; (2) average Medicare out-of-pocket expenses (including Part B premiums, private "Medigap" insurance, deductibles, and uncovered services) already took 23 percent of the average income of Americans over sixty-five and were expected to rise; (3) employers' health costs were rising and, consequently, the percentage of firms offering any insurance coverage had steadily fallen from nearly 68 percent in 2000 to 60 percent in 2005; (4) workers' health insurance premiums were rising faster than their wages, and the total cost of an insurance policy for a family was approaching $14,565 annually; (5) medical bills were the cause of half of all personal bankruptcies—and more than 75 percent who went bankrupt had been insured at the beginning of a bankrupting illness; (6) most Americans were totally unaware of the costs of long-term care and unaware that such costs were not covered by Medicare.

AARP's focus groups and surveys revealed a surprising paradox: Americans didn't see health care as a consumer good to shop for but as a fundamental right that no one should be denied. This was very close to the views of Canadians and Europeans. Yet the research also confirmed Americans' abiding mistrust of government (except as a watchdog) and their resentment toward unflattering comparisons with other nations—notwithstanding the success of *Sicko,* Michael Moore's documentary that indicted America's health care system while praising that of France and even Cuba.

Flawed as it is, Americans still think they have the best system. Therefore, "Talk about improving the system, not overhauling it," instructed Rother. "And present it as an *American* solution." Americans preferred private-public, not government solutions. Hence, the terms *comprehensive* and *universal* were to be avoided.

The high costs of care and the limited access to it were market issues that were clearly understood as problems. However, many Americans believed it was possible to address these without spending more money. Therefore, reformers had to stress that any new taxes would be limited.

Medicare remained popular, said Rother, though it was both amusing and infuriating that some citizens didn't recognize it as a government program. "They'll say, 'Keep government out of my Medicare'" Rother joked. Cost reductions in Medicare had to be seen as part of broader reforms.

Quality and *affordable* were among the "words that work," according to AARP research. "Access to quality health care" was a magic slogan. So were the phrases "patient-centered care" and "freedom and flexibility." The term *consumer* did not test well, nor did social science jargon like *systems* or *systemwide* or *disease management.* People in the AARP studies did understand the concept and importance of prevention as long as it was presented in terms of personal action (such as cancer screenings).

Finally—and in line with Bill Novelli's increasing emphasis on generational outreach—the AARP PowerPoint blueprint presented the normative maxim that "intergenerational support is the mark of a civilized society." In discussing health care reform, the benefits to family and all generations had to be stressed.

The PowerPoint slides shifted to the red-and-white color scheme and bulleted goals of "Divided We Fail." Among them:

- Access to affordable, quality health care, including prescription drugs, in a way that costs will not burden future generations
- Wellness and preventive care priorities should include changes in personal behavior, such as diet and exercise
- All children should be covered
- Health information technology must be improved and updated
- Defense of Medicare
- Support of innovative state health reforms
- Provide choice and flexibility in long-term care

As was often the case when Rother spoke publicly about the Divided We Fail plan, the first questioner challenged Rother about why AARP wasn't pressing the case for government-financed, single-payer "Medicare for all"—similar to the Canadian health care system. As he was used to doing, Rother cited American's long-standing mistrust of government but also hinted that the goals of "Divided We Fail" involved substantial bargaining and compromise in order to entice the Business Roundtable into the AARP-SEIU alliance. AARP's strenuous efforts to be bipartisan carried a price. Indeed.

As this blueprint was put into action, the Divided We Fail alliance initially helped raise political awareness about the need for major health care reform. AARP members wearing bright red "Divided We Fail" T-shirts were highly visible during the early presidential primaries—raising public awareness and pushing the candidates to talk about health care.

In early 2008, AARP California rallied to support Governor Arnold Schwarzenegger's major policy push for state health care mandates. AARP's Bill Novelli flew out to join Schwarzenegger in the opening ceremony for the campaign. But Schwarzenegger's ambitious blueprint collapsed in the legislature partly because the issue of health care reform in California and elsewhere was upstaged by the collapsing bubble in real estate prices, a summer spike in energy and food prices, and, of course, the autumn stock market meltdown.

Between February and July 2008, according to a Pew Research Center poll, the percentage of Americans ranking "prices" as the "most important economic problem facing the nation" nearly doubled from 24 to 45 percent. Concern over "gasoline/oil/energy" led this concern, nearly tripling from 11 to 38 percent; cost-of-living worries jumped from 5 to 9 percent; but concern over health care and medical prices fell from 9 to 2 percent.[48] The autumn stock market crash further eclipsed almost all other noneconomic issues.

Still, AARP kept pouring money into the Divided We Fail campaign via very visible television and full-page magazine advertising. Such persistence kept health care reform on the political agenda and paved the way for the new Obama administration to make the issue its top priority. Even after the 2008 elections, AARP's advocacy network urged members to again send e-mails to the new Congress and president-elect, reminding them of their campaign pledges on health care reform. The e-mail barrage was followed up by face-to-face meetings between congressional representatives and AARP members (in red "Divided We Fail" T-shirts).

As will be discussed in greater detail in the next chapter, the Divided We Fail campaign's core emphases on "access, affordability, and quality" (as well as the more specific tactics and goals outlined in the AARP PowerPoint presentation) were picked up by other lobbying groups and incorporated into the language of the congressional bills that ultimately became the signed legislation. The 2008 elections also focused professional, public, and news media interest in the nation's cultural diversity and changing demographics. A 2008 census bureau study advanced the date when whites would be less than 50 percent of the nation's population from 2050 to 2042. The surge in minority populations was becoming especially evident among youth.[49] These changes were embodied in the emergence of a postboomer political wave that powered election of the first biracial "postboomer" Democratic Party presidential candidate, Senator Barack Obama.

Once again, though, AARP was ahead of the curve.

AARP DEEPENS ITS DIVERSITY MISSION

African rhythms pounded out by a local African American folk drumming group greeted about 850 registrants for the AARP "Diversity and Aging in the 21st Century" conference as they filed into the main ballroom at the Los Angeles Bonaventure Hotel. The three-day conference in late June 2007 was designed to highlight AARP's escalating interest in the nation's rapid demographic change and burgeoning cultural diversity. Many of AARP's board of directors were present, as were Bill Novelli and most of his management team. In 2009, AARP would select A. Barry Rand, a former executive at Xerox and Avis Car Rental, as its first African American CEO.

Affirmative action and other efforts to increase female and minority representation have long been woven into AARP's organizational procedures and culture. Since 1998, there have been two black female AARP presidents. Retired or still employed African American teachers and public employees are visible constituencies at AARP conferences. Diversity is a criterion in selecting AARP's board members, its officers, and its staff and is evident in feature stories and advertisements in AARP's publications. The organization celebrates Black History Month, Hispanic Heritage Month, Gay Pride Month, and so on. A special Hispanic-themed conference in Puerto Rico 2007 sold out its fifteen thousand capacity. During its fiftieth anniversary year, 2008, AARP distributed $1 million in Legacy Awards to (mostly minority and/or inner-city) high school programs demonstrating "a commitment to connect generations and foster greater civic engagement among students and their communities."[50] AARP has become a major sponsor for a range of ethnic and gender special interest conferences ranging from the annual NAACP conference to smaller events such as

"It's About Time: LGBT [Lesbian, Gay, Bisexual Transgender] Aging in a Changing World."

Diversity and the Divided We Fail campaign were constantly coupled at the "Diversity and Aging in the 21st Century" conference. Thus, in his official welcome, AARP chief diversity officer Percil Stanford was quick to get on message by declaring, "We need to work together— or 'Divided We Fail.'"

"We are all part of change," Stanford explained, warning that "diversity may be difficult to accept, for it means sharing or giving up of power and resources." Stanford ritually invoked AARP's founder, Ethel Percy Andrus, describing how proud the retired school principal would have been of the dedication ceremony he had just attended at the brand-new Ethel Percy Andrus Center for the Performing Arts at inner-city L.A.'s Abraham Lincoln High School. "All the kids there had AARP T-shirts," he happily observed, and concluded, to a wave of applause, that "we need to give every kid [in the country] an AARP T-shirt!"

Board of directors president Erik F. Olsen, a former dentist and for fifteen years the director of the giant Delta Dental insurance corporation, quickly linked diversity and health care reform by mentioning that Delta Dental had worked with Cesar Chavez to obtain affordable health care for farmworkers. "Throughout much of my life, America looked like a microcosm of Europe," said Olson. "Today, we are a microcosm of the world." To remain a leader, AARP must embrace diversity. Olson then launched into discourse on the nation's health care problems and the goals of "Divided We Fail."

L.A.'s first Hispanic mayor, Antonio Villaraigosa, extended his official conference welcome, emphasizing L.A.'s historically global nature. He described its origins as a mostly Mexican-majority city in the mid-1800s that became majority Anglo during the twentieth century and is today again becoming a predominantly Latino city—the latter statement eliciting scattered applause. He stressed the mutual dependence of younger immigrants and the elderly. Villaraigosa joked that the full impact of his identity as a grandfather hit home when AARP asked him to be on the cover of its monthly magazine. On behalf of the city, he accepted a diversity sculpture from AARP presented by CEO Bill Novelli, who proudly observed that Villaraigosa was wearing an AARP "Divided We Fail" pin. (The next day, another celebrity speaker, the civil rights activist, former congressman, and NAACP president Julian Bond, publicly signed a "Divided We Fail" pledge that Novelli promised to publicly display at AARP headquarters. AARP has also become a primary sponsor for NAACP's national conferences.)

The two-day "Diversity in the 21st Century" gathering featured a variety of lectures, panels, and workshops on topics ranging from the changing markets for age fifty-plus Americans to growing ethnic diversity in elderly communities, aging gay men and lesbians, aging in prison, long-term care in a diverse society, and reshaping the images of aging. AARP president-elect Jennie Chin Hansen chaired a roundtable discussion for reporters from ethnic media sources. Luncheons, a lavish evening reception-and-multicultural buffet, and a tour de force one-woman show by the writer-performer Anna Deavere Smith were underwritten by official sponsors United Health Group and the giant California Endowment.

I encountered Erik Olsen and AARP's chief operating officer Tom Nelson standing together in the middle of the bustling outdoor reception-buffet. The two white men seemed to be deeply pondering the sights and sounds of their three-day immersion in L.A.'s ethnic and cultural landscape. "We're taking this all in," said Olsen. "Now we've got to back and figure out how to process and act on all this."

CHAPTER SIX

AARP Turns Fifty

The Battle for Health Care Reform

Like many of the boomers whom it was courting, AARP itself turned fifty in 2008 and celebrated with an enhanced "Life @ 50+" celebration in Washington, D.C., just after Labor Day. The organization's multigenerational outreach was heralded in the conference theme of "Generations Connecting to Change." Throughout the giant Washington, D.C., Convention Center, Ethel Percy Andrus's portraits, life story, and favorite slogans ("To serve, not be served") were everywhere. The long-deceased female founder's name was most frequently invoked during opening day welcoming speeches by AARP officials and by a company of actors portraying the history of AARP.

This would be Bill Novelli's last performance as ringmaster for the annual event. He skillfully mixed Andrus's simple legacy with his own increasingly ambitious and extensive AARP agenda. He especially highlighted the conference themes of an increased focus on younger generations and on global aging and international alliances. (There was a hospitality suite in the convention center for AARP's global affiliates.) He also hailed the efforts of the "Divided We Fail" health care reform alliance. (The hybrid donkey-elephant logo was a ubiquitous feature in the convention center).

The main event at this fiftieth-anniversary celebration was a star-studded gala in front of the Lincoln Memorial on the afternoon of the conference's opening day. The event featured several well-known speakers, including the NASCAR celebrity driver Richard Petty, the country singer Wynona Rider, the movie star Sally Field, and the daughter of Martin Luther King. But though official conference total registration was approximately 27,500, only about 4,500 people attended the Lincoln Memorial ceremonies. Approximately half of those who braved the muggy heat were conscripts—employees drafted from AARP's vast D.C. headquarters, readily identifiable by their red "AARP 50th Anniversary" T-shirts. Transportation was another problem. The event was nearly a mile from the nearest Washington Metro subway stop, and there were long lines for chartered buses at the convention center. Hundreds of chairs on the hot, sunny north side of the long reflecting pool remained empty—most of the audience favored sitting or standing on the shadier south side. Some of the presentations were temporarily drowned out by commercial jet aircraft passing low overhead on their landing paths into Reagan National Airport, just across the Potomac. Despite the heat, disappointing attendance, and descending aircraft, however, the planners were very lucky that the outdoor ceremony took place only forty hours before the remnants of Hurricane Hanna hit the capital with high winds and torrents of rain.

The storm's arrival on Saturday morning did not dampen conference goers' enthusiasm for a satellite teleconference with Democratic presidential candidate Barack Obama at 8:30 a.m. About four thousand AARP members packed the convention center ballroom to listen to Obama give a short speech and then field questions from Bill Novelli via a satellite uplink. (At the conclusion, many in the audience enthusiastically burst into a rhythmic campaign chant, "O-bam-a! O-bam-a!") A few hours later, a similar satellite interchange with Republican candidate John McCain drew only a few hundred people; indeed, the crowd was so sparse and placid that AARP conference staff pleaded with the audience to move closer to the front of the ballroom to give to McCain and the television networks recording the event the illusion of a larger gathering.

This obvious political tilt was an embarrassment to an organization striving to present itself as a nonpartisan microcosm for all of fifty-plus America. And the conference crowds illustrated other continuing demographic imbalances as well.

First, the Life @ 50+ audiences illustrated that an aging society is an increasingly female society. Though AARP's official membership is 55 percent female, perhaps two-thirds of those attending the Washington, D.C., Life @ 50+ were women. Single men seemed very scarce. There were many married couples. But what was striking were the large numbers of single, divorced, or widowed women—almost always in the company of one or two others. Many to whom I spoke evidently viewed the three-day conference as an opportunity for a "girls' night out." It was mostly women who streamed into the aisles and rushed to the front of the cavernous, convention center hall when (on their respective concert nights) both Paul Simon and members of the band Chicago invited the audience to come down and "party" in front of the stage. Clusters of women were even more apparent at the Life @ 50+ music-and-dance clubs, which (as at previous conventions) featured classic rock, Latin, and blues/soul entertainment. (Rock band numbers that featured line dancing—requiring no partners—filled the ballroom dance floor with women.)

Second, AARP continues to struggle with ethnic and cultural diversity issues. Though influenced by the Washington, D.C., setting (with its majority African American population), the conference's demographics illustrated the gap between the nation's urban demographic landscape and AARP's still overwhelmingly white (89 percent) and middle-class registered membership. Yet AARP's marked emphasis on ethnic diversity in conference keynote speakers, lecture topics, and entertainment produced the paradoxical results typical of such efforts throughout American society: an uneasy mix of both unity and separatism.

The closing keynote speakers Quincy Jones and Maya Angelou (the latter a perennial Life @ 50+ favorite) provided a sense of warm, color-transcending unity. (This may have been because—as both of them noted—they had received instructions to avoid political commentary.) The conference hall was crowded, and during question-and-answer sessions many whites gushed effusively that they were honored to be "in their presence." (One white inner-city high school teacher choked back sobs when he asked Angelou's advice on dealing with burnout and the desire to quit.) Yet the audiences attending the three major evening concerts provided reminders of persistent, deep cultural preferences. The Thursday night concert featuring Chaka Khan and Natalie Cole drew the most African Americans; there were far fewer blacks at the Friday night concert by the all-white rock band Chicago; and perhaps 90 percent of those attending the concluding Saturday evening concert by 1960s-era singer Paul Simon were white. (That audience witnessed an impressive postconcert fiftieth-anniversary light show featuring showers of golden confetti shot from mock cannons.)

In his last year as CEO, Bill Novelli held fast to his formula for building a more ethnically inclusive, multigenerational, big-tent AARP by emphasizing common values and life concerns. He explained to me,

> When I first came here, the question was still on the table as to whether AARP could appeal to baby boomers and recruit them as members—while still staying loyal and relevant to older members. A third of our members are now boomers, so the answer is yes. The differences between boomers and older people are more superficial, surface characteristics. Their wants are somewhat different. But when you get down to the level of needs, everyone needs health and health care and they need long-term financial security. Then, when you get down to the level of values, all generations are the same: they want a better world for their children and grandchildren; they want to leave the world a better place and to leave a legacy. These are common values, and that's what we've built upon.[1]

The 1.6 million-member "Divided We Fail" health care reform alliance was just such a multigroup vehicle for "connecting generations for change." The campaign's emphasis on health care access, affordability, and quality for all Americans broadened the organization's "brand" appeal and rebutted critics' charges that AARP was a "greedy geezer" lobby. The alliance with business organizations and failure to even mention government-funded health care system (similar to Canada's) blunted conservative accusations that AARP was merely a Democratic front for big-government programs. Finally, Divided We Fail's focus on total health care reform tried to shift the focus away from Medicare and the popular definition of the elderly as "problems." It made everyone a stakeholder in change.

As mentioned in the previous chapter, by the end of 2008, the Divided We Fail campaign could be credited with helping to keep the issue of health care reform publicly visible and not entirely eclipsed by the economic crises. Divided We Fail unquestionably articulated and advanced the "access-affordability-quality" themes eventually incorporated into the title of the 2010 Democrat-backed comprehensive health care reform legislation: the Patient Protection and Affordable Care Act (PPACA). Indeed, by the end of 2008, AARP's Divided We Fail Web page proclaimed that more than two-thirds of new Congress members (though comparatively few Republicans) registered agreement with the goals of Divided We Fail. And the Obama White House Agenda page on health care reform, Social Security, and several other issues reflected substantial agreement with AARP.

And so the man that Alan Simpson had sarcastically dubbed "the Wizard of Oz" had successfully maneuvered AARP into a primary role in the most important entitlement debates since Social Security and Medicare were founded. But this mission would not be an easy one. A. Barry Rand, Novelli's successor and the first African American to head AARP, must continue to juggle many competing interests and navigate some of the most turbulent political waters ever encountered by the age fifty-plus organization.

"A new era in Washington has begun!" was Bill Novelli's 2009 New Year's e-mail greeting to AARP members. "Our time is now!"

Or so it seemed.

A NONPARTISAN CENTER-LEFT AGENDA

After the 2008 election, AARP's Grassroots America advocacy unit notified its six million members to e-mail or write their congressional representatives and President Obama to take action on four major issues: (1) making health care more affordable, (2) protecting and strengthening Social Security, (3) safeguarding and improving pensions and retirement savings plans, and (4) keeping age discrimination out of the workplace.[2]

These goals were general, bland, and almost apolitical. Most Americans would likely agree with them without a second thought. Indeed, before the 2009 health care reform battles, most Americans and even a majority of AARP members may have been largely unaware of AARP's politics. (*New York Times* "Generation B" columnist Michael Winerip admitted to me that he utilized data from AARP but knew little about their politics.[3] So did *Examiner.com*'s baby boomer columnist Paul Briand.)[4]

For those who have been culturally and politically attuned, however, AARP's publications, conferences, advocacy campaigns, Web page, and other aspects of its public face reveal an organizational culture and politics that is moderately liberal—largely a reflection of the culture and ideology of the upper-middle and professional classes discussed at length in chapter 3. This worldview is built upon an often tacit, taken-for-granted acceptance of globalization, mass immigration, multiculturalism, and the belief that the nation's economy, growing age/class/ethnic schisms, and civic culture can be "managed" in a bipartisan fashion. AARP's publications and other media appear to reflect the culture and mores of the Beltway leadership elite and its house organs, the *New*

York Times and the *Washington Post.* (AARP's magazine cover stories and convention events also regularly feature Hollywood celebrities, many of whom are perceived to be liberal.) And, as illustrated at the end of the previous chapter, AARP vigorously celebrates diversity, including gay/lesbian/transgender lifestyles and rights. (In 2009 the AARP Web page had a major feature on the fortieth anniversary of the 1969 Greenwich Village Stonewall riots, a response to a New York City police raid on a gay tavern historically regarded as the trigger of the modern gay rights movement.)

In a July 2010 interview, Novelli told me that one of his achievements as AARP's CEO was to make it a more "pragmatic, middle-of-the-road organization." Perhaps. Politically, it is difficult to distinguish most of AARP's "nonpartisan" policy positions from those of moderate Democrats. Under its 501(c)(4) IRS status, AARP may address issues affecting older Americans through a variety of means, including lobbying efforts at the state and national governmental level, but it is not supposed to support, oppose, or donate to political parties or candidates. Yet AARP's e-mail advocacy list of six million and its Congresswatch Web site seem far more positively attuned to Democratic congressional or White House proposals. In early 2008, AARP lobbied for expansion of the States Children's Health Insurance Program (SCHIP), which passed Congress but was vetoed by President Bush. (In January 2009, President Obama signed an identical act.) In the fall of 2008, AARP utilized its grassroots lobbying network to mobilize 110,000 e-mails to Congress members to support the Troubled Asset Relief Program (TARP) bank rescue legislation.[5] In January 2009, the advocacy network rallied its e-mail troops to support the economic stimulus package.

Two-thirds of AARP's 2008 Congressional Awards recipients were Democrats.[6] And while AARP did not directly endorse any of the 2008 presidential candidates, *AARP Magazine's* three-way comparison of Barack Obama, John McCain, and AARP on key issues constituted a de facto Obama recommendation. On commitment to ending gridlock, ensuring Social Security (without diverting funds into individual accounts), establishing automatic payroll deductions for IRAs, preserving Medicare, and enacting health care reform, AARP and candidate Obama were in full agreement. McCain refused to participate. (His strategists no doubt sensed a trap. Had McCain agreed with AARP on more than one or two issues, he would have been pilloried by GOP conservatives; and if he appeared weak on Social Security or Medicare, he might have lost the senior vote—as it turned out, the only age group that he carried.)[7]

By 2010, AARP's Web page featured a "Yourvote" section that enabled interested members and nonmembers alike to use zip-code focusing to compare AARP's policy positions issues with those of local congressional and statewide office candidates. As with the Obama-McCain comparisons, AARP did not explicitly endorse candidates that agreed with its positions—though the implicit intent was fairly obvious.

ARP's officials and researchers tend to deny its center-left political persona altogether or to state that, in any case, public perceptions of its alleged liberalism have little effect on attracting new members. Their internal research indicates that the political views of their membership reflect those of the general electorate.[8] Still, AARP seemed unprepared for the gathering storm that their support for Democratic-sponsored health care reform (see below) would elicit from an apparently wide range of members.

AARP's long-term tilt toward Democratic Party positions was becoming risky on several fronts. First, it jeopardized the "nonpartisan trust" brand vital to AARP's products-and-services enterprises. Second, consistent support of Democratic objectives gave credence to Republicans' and conservatives' complaints that AARP promoted a partisan political agenda that, along with its insurance and financial sales, called into question its non-profit 504(c) status. Third, this somewhat left-of-center stance still failed to please committed liberal Democrats who continued to complain that AARP was primarily a money-making machine that too readily sold out political for commercial interests— such as the refusal to promote a Canadian-style single-payer health care agenda.[9] Finally, support of Democratic initiatives tied AARP to the short- or long-term success or failure of those efforts. Thus, though AARP endorsement of the 2008 TARP legislation and the 2009 Obama Democrats' stimulus package, budget, and health care bills proved successful in the short term, the organization would be held responsible by millions of members if the economy did not recover or—especially—if there were reductions in Medicare services.

"WARRIOR BRAND" MEETS A "SENIOR MINI-MUTINY"

"We own Social Security and Medicare," an AARP board member told me emphatically in mid-2008. But this same board member admitted an increasingly obvious policy stance open to compromise and cutbacks—usually signaled by official calls to "preserve Social Security and Medicare for future generations." But how great the compromise and how stern the limits? This was soon to be tested.

As the health care reform battle lines took shape in the spring of 2009, AARP's new president, A. Barry Rand, and his staff donned their warrior-brand armor. Rand emphasized the organization's interests in enhancing and preserving Medicare. The first major goal was to close the gap in Medicare's supplemental drug coverage gap known as the "donut hole." A second aim was to create a Medicare "transitional benefit," for supportive services needed after hospitalization. A third AARP priority was to ensure that younger members, aged fifty to sixty-four, had a "choice of affordable health care" (though AARP did not advocate a proposal once floated by President Clinton—lowering the eligibility age for Medicare).[10]

The goal of at least partially closing the Medicare prescription coverage drug "donut hole" was achieved in July. In a White House ceremony with Barry Rand at his side, President Obama proudly announced that AARP and the pharmaceutical industry—aided by Congress and the Obama White House—had reached an agreement to lower drug prices 50 percent for Medicare recipients who were in the donut-hole coverage gap. (AARP lost a separate battle for lower drug prices when the Congress health care reform plan included a pharmaceutical industry request for twelve-year market exclusivity for branded biotechnology drugs—no competition from cheaper generic brands during that period.)[11] But AARP's other stated health care reform goals of cutting the growth of health care costs through rational measurement, management, and elimination of "wasteful" Medicare practices began to arouse suspicions of redistribution and rationing.[12]

At the beginning of President Barack Obama's new term, the AARP Web site featured a YouTube video clip of Bill Novelli and President Obama publicly agreeing about the priority of comprehensive, cost-effective health care at a White House Fiscal Responsibility Summit. The video drew mostly critical comments from the Right and from the Left. Conservatives were suspicious of "socialism"; liberals pleaded for a single-payer, government-financed system like Canada's.

One posted comment in particular signaled AARP's strategic dilemma regarding boomers and older Americans: whether to defend and maximize Medicare benefits or accept (tacitly) a measure of "redistribution," compromise, and cutbacks: "Why cut Medicare benefits so we can give insurance to the uninsured? Why charge our elderly for the problem? This is entitlement redistribution. Pure Medicare doesn't cover nearly enough of our medical expenses. When is AARP going to speak out and help protect Senior benefits?"[13] This message embodied AARP's worst nightmare: that significant numbers of the fifty-plus population perceived comprehensive health care reform as a zero-sum game, an "us-versus-them" battle that jeopardized an already underfunded Medicare system by redistributing resources to younger Americans, including (many suspected) illegal immigrants.

In the spring and early summer, AARP continued to champion its more general Divided We Fail agenda while avoiding explicit endorsement of emerging House and Senate health care reform bills. Initially, the organization tried to have it both ways. On the one hand,

on its www.keepmedicarefair.org Web site, the organization priori-
tized stabilizing Medicare premium increases and adding services.
But AARP also started a new Web site, HealthActionNow.org, invit-
ing visitors to sign a petition urging swift congressional action, along
with a blog to share personal stories illustrating problems with the
current system.

The line between AARP's coveted "nonpartisan" commercial trust
brand and its advocacy "warrior" image dissolved as it became more
entangled in defending Democrats' reform proposals. Two developments proved especially troublesome.

First, in midsummer 2009 one of the major drafts of health care
reform legislation, congressional health care reform bill H.R. 3200,
contained a proposal to finance health care reform in part through
more than five hundred billion dollars in reduced future spending on
Medicare and Medicaid. This feature endured and became part of the
final PPACA.

The proposed spending reduction immediately raised cries of
rationing and redistribution and accusations that health care reform
would be accomplished at the expense of older Americans. Talk of
"death panels" began to surface, and the flow of angry e-mails to the
AARP Web site became a torrent, with heated accusations that the
organization was selling out its members—evidence of what a *New York
Times* reporter termed a "senior mini-mutiny."

Second, President Obama began invoking AARP's name in promoting health care reform. Indeed, on July 28, 2009, President Obama and
AARP visually merged. The president stood in front a large AARP
logo for more than an hour during a Webcast "tele-townhall forum" in
which Obama fielded health care reform questions from telephone call-
ers and a small, live audience. Casual viewers of forum excerpts on the
nightly newscasts or on the Web easily presumed that AARP "backed"
the president with more than just their logo. Indeed, the president himself presumed as much two weeks later when he publicly declared: "We
have the AARP on board because they know this is a good deal for

our seniors." In the same setting he later denied Medicare cutbacks, saying, "AARP would not be endorsing a bill if it was undermining Medicare, okay?"[14]

The news media also fueled perceptions that AARP had endorsed the Democratic health care reform bills. For example, on July 26, 2009, *New York Times* editorial writers concluded a two-thousand-word lead editorial on health care reform by suggesting an implicit AARP endorsement: "The AARP, the main lobby for older Americans, has praised the emerging bills and thrown its weight behind the cause. All of this suggests to us that the great majority of Americans—those with insurance and those without—would benefit from health care reform."[15]

AARP quickly issued an official denial of any such explicit endorsement. Yet on the same day as the official denial, AARP policy director John Rother blurred this denial somewhat when he responded to a question from MSNBC's Rachel Maddow about opponents' scare tactics. "We have read every page of the bills and we've concluded that the bills proposed in Congress would be good for seniors," Rother assured viewers. "[There is] nothing to be scared about in the actual legislation."[16]

AARP's efforts to defend emerging health care reform proposals on its Web page continued to be met with member responses that were nearly always overwhelmingly negative:

> The fact that AARP would support this program is ludicrous. This is not only a poor choice for the country, but it is a more serious concern for seniors. Who do you think government rationing will affect first and foremost? Of course the answer is seniors. Do the right thing rather than your typical left wing stance. Get the liberal blinders off and look at this for what it is. Continued failure to take a balanced approach to issues leaves me no choice to make the decision to not renew my membership.[17]

> After 23 years I have just cancelled my membership in AARP. Does the management of AARP actually think they are providing a benefit or service to AARP members by conspiring with the Obama administration to finance the current healthcare debacle on the backs of senior citizens?

Given the way the administration is handling this issue, it is impossible to know what in hell the law will be, or what effect it will have, except to decrease coverage for living seniors, and assist in accelerating their "end of life." I'm waiting for some bright Washington "beanhead" to suggest that the problem can be resolved much more quickly (even before the end of Obama's first term) and efficiently by simply getting rid of 40 million pesky senior citizens! After all, we and our crooked doctors are to blame. And just think of the jobs it would create in the funeral industry![18]

AARP's leaders quickly moved into damage control. CEO Barry Rand responded sharply to press reports that members of Congress were eyeing even larger Medicare cuts over the next decade than those originally proposed in the House bill, H.R. 3200. "AARP cannot support any efforts to target Medicare beneficiaries for increased cost-sharing or other benefit cuts," warned Rand. Other national and regional officers went into action. A raking critique of AARP, "Obamacare Could Kill AARP," by Mark Tapscott in *WashingtonExaminer.com* was answered there in a matter of hours by the AARP vice president, Drew Nannis, in "AARP: Setting the Record Straight."[19] Through press releases and on radio and television, AARP's articulate policy director John Rother tried to clarify AARP positions and jousted in print and on talk shows with prominent critics of the proposals.[20]

During the August congressional recess, AARP tried to debunk health care reform "myths" mushrooming at local town hall meetings—including one raucous Dallas AARP forum where local AARP officials simply walked out. (A video of the meeting received wide viewing on YouTube.) A one-page document entitled "Myths vs. Facts" on the AARP Web site denied that health care reform would (1) be socialized medicine, (2) result in rationed care, (3) hurt Medicare, or (4) be too expensive. In fine print, there was an admission of improving Medicare's quality and "eliminating billions in waste."

AARP also launched a multi-million-dollar series of radio and television ads. Throughout the health care reform battles, it was actively lobbying Congress members and undoubtedly played a role in a forcing

White House reversal of an early concession to the pharmaceutical lobby to continue the Bush-era ban on Medicare's ability to bargain with drug companies over prices. Members of the AARP "Divided We Fail" initiative as well as those registered for AARP Grassroots America were regularly updated through e-mail messages—often containing links to congressional offices.

Most Americans simply did not share the urgency felt by AARP, Congress, and the White House. Nearly 80 percent did *not* believe that there was a crisis in U.S. health care, nor did they believe that benefits would accrue to them personally or reduce overall costs—according to a Gallup poll. Most favored some government involvement in health care, but fewer than half favored a government-run health care system.[21] Debate over health care reform became so intense that thousands of e-mails overloaded the House of Representatives' Web site.[22]

Nevertheless, into the late summer of 2009, senior citizens continued to assert that health care reform would come at their expense, a perception reinforced by the *Washington Post's* Ceci Connolly. "From the raw numbers, it appears seniors are the net losers under bills approved by three House committees last week. . . . The legislation trims $563 billion out of Medicare's growth rate over the next 10 years, while pumping in about $350 billion."[23]

AARP and other health care reform supporters confronted an unwelcome and growing public opinion age split toward health care reform: generally, Americans over age fifty opposed it; those under fifty supported it.[24] More specifically, according to a Pew Research Center survey, only 29 percent of those over age sixty-five supported health care reform versus 44 percent of those aged eighteen to twenty-nine. Forty-five percent of Older Boomers (aged fifty to sixty-four) favored the plan but only 34 percent of Younger Boomers and Generation X (aged thirty to forty-nine). A third of whites favored the plan, while half of blacks did. Thirty-five percent of those with incomes above $75,000 were favorably inclined versus 44 percent with incomes less than $30,000. The most decisive variable was political identification: 61

percent of Democrats were favorable versus 12 percent of Republicans and 34 percent of independents.[25]

HEALTH CARE REFORMERS SIDESTEP
IMMIGRATION POLICY LANDMINES

A substantial number of the angry e-mails cascading onto the AARP Web site (and also the sites of the major news media) indicated that average citizens were much quicker than elites to detect a potential redistribution of health care services from older, largely white Americans to younger immigrant populations. Democrats and AARP found themselves trying to straddle the emerging age/class/ethnic triple divide discussed in previous chapters.

More than half of respondents to an August 2009 NBC News poll agreed that health care reform would ultimately give health care coverage to illegal immigrants.[26] (But it took the *Wall Street Journal* nearly a month to offer a small front-page story entitled "Illegal Immigration Enters the Health-Care Debate."[27] A week later, the *Los Angeles Times* more directly confronted the topic in an editorial titled "Illegal Immigrants Debate Could Potentially Block Reform.")[28]

Indeed, before and after the ultimate, narrow passage of the legislation, working- and middle-class whites over age fifty remained skeptical of health care and, increasingly, the rest of the Obama administration's agenda. In October 2009 Ronald Brownstein, analyzing a National Journal/Heartland America poll, noticed that only 40 percent of whites supported health care reform compared to 75 percent of non-whites.[29] *Huffington Post* political editor Thomas Edsall bitterly blamed a racial and demographic divide for almost dooming health care reform: "The harsh reality is many [white] voters consider the health care bill a multibillion-dollar transfer of taxpayer money to the uninsured, a population disproportionately, although by no means exclusively, made up of the poor, African Americans, Latinos, single parents and the long-term unemployed."[30]

But older and many white Americans' suspicions of this broad-scale social change were grounded in a measure of common sense. There was the inevitable realization that the inclusion of forty-seven million uninsured into a vast new system of health insurance and services while not increasing overall costs (keeping health care expenditures "revenue neutral") would necessarily result in substantial changes. This meant some degree of rationing and redistribution of services away from those currently using a disproportionate share of health care costs and services: senior citizens, especially those in their last year of life. (And despite the jeers of pundits, many citizens correctly perceived that illegal immigrants—21 percent of the uninsured—would eventually gain access to the system, especially if the Obama White House made good on its public proclamations for immigration reform that would include a "pathway to citizenship.")

These patterns of skepticism persisted after passage of health care reform. A Gallup poll found that only 20 percent of whites thought health care reform would benefit them, though a majority admitted that the enacted legislation would help uninsured and low-income families.[31] A *Wall Street Journal*/NBC News poll found Obama concurrently losing support among Americans making $50,000 to $75,000, "a predominantly white group over age 50 but not yet retired" (in other words, working-and middle-class Older Boomers).[32] Indeed there was some indication that sentiments for repealing "ObamaCare" were rising, perhaps spurred by the controversy generated when Arizona enacted a new law to identify illegal immigrants in 2010. The pollster Peter Brown immediately recognized a familiar age-class-culture division: "Like Affirmative Action, Arizona Law Splits Elites and the Public."[33]

IN AARP WE (STILL) TRUST

As the last member of the U.S. House of Representatives to speak just before the climatic March 9, 2010, vote on the Senate version of what would become the PPACA, Speaker of the House Nancy Pelosi very publicly saluted AARP for its consistent support and specifically for its endorsement of "cracking down on fraud and waste in Medicare and strengthening Medicare for today's seniors and future generations of seniors." Indeed, Pelosi reportedly credited AARP and Andy Stern's Service Employees International Union (SEIU) as the two primary organizational forces behind the bill. Yet despite such notable identification with a polarizing cause, AARP received little notice in the mainstream press—critical or otherwise.

In mid-October of 2009, the *Christian Science Monitor* quoted AARP executive vice president Nancy LeaMond that the intensifying health care reform battle had become something of a "roller derby."[34] A more critical *Washington Post* analysis in late October revisited the organization's dual identity and potential conflict of interest as both "reform advocate and insurance salesman" and noted the high pay of AARP executives.[35] A *New York Times* report suggested a generational battle and "mini-mutiny" within AARP over perceptions that the young (through mandatory insurance enrollment) and the old (through reductions in projected Medicare spending) were going to be sacrificed to obtain reduced insurance rates for the middle-aged.[36]

But AARP officials were getting comparatively good news on how their coveted "trust" image was faring. An AARP sample survey of its members that indicated that, indeed, when informed about congressional bills' key provisions and AARP support, 39 percent "strongly supported" the plan and another 24 percent "somewhat supported" it. AARP was also gratified to discover that more than 80 percent of survey respondents indicated that they trusted AARP's position on health care because "as a non-partisan organization AARP is an independent voice fighting for the best interest of people over 50." These findings had been foreshadowed the previous month by a National Public Radio/Kaiser Family Foundation/Harvard School of Public Health survey. AARP was ranked first among seven health reform interest groups (by nearly a 20-point margin over second-place Consumers Union) by Democrats and Independents, who indicated confidence that AARP would "recommend the right thing for the country on health care." (For Republicans, AARP tied with "health insurance companies.")[37]

Fortified by these results, on December 19, 2009, Nancy LeaMond posted a letter to the AARP Web site that she had sent to all U.S. senators urging them to vote for cloture on the Senate's PPACA. "Given the importance of bringing this debate to a close and securing timely Senate passage of health care legislation, AARP has designated the cloture motion . . . a key vote. As part of our ongoing effort to let our members know of action taken on key issues we will be informing them of how their Senators vote on this cloture motion." Members enrolled in AARP's Grassroots America campaign were updated on key votes and urged to contact their congressional representatives.

A mid-November Rasmussen telephone voter survey, however, found more mixed views of AARP. Fifty-three percent of all respondents had at least a somewhat favorable view of AARP—but nearly 40 percent had an unfavorable view. Eighty percent of Democrats had a favorable perception of AARP as opposed to 58 percent of Republicans and 39 percent of independents—but nearly 48 percent of the latter had a negative assessment. Ironically, the organization registered higher support with survey respondents under age thirty (60 percent) than those over age fifty (49 percent). When survey respondents were informed of AARP's support of the Democratic health care plan, favorable opinion of AARP fell from 53 to 43 percent. The good news for AARP's leaders was that Rasmussen survey respondents had a somewhat confused, nonpartisan perception of AARP's politics: 38 percent thought AARP was generally supportive of Democrats, 8 percent thought it favored Republicans, 36 percent thought it was equally supportive of both parties, and 17 percent weren't sure.[38]

These generally positive polling data sharply contrasted with escalating criticism of AARP in the blogosphere and in newspaper letters to the editor. Especially as AARP's support of Democratic health reform initiatives became more widely known, almost all of the blogosphere political commentary waxed critical, often ending with a declaration of rejecting AARP literature or with a promise to tear up membership cards. (One blogger archly dubbed himself a member of the "New" AARP: Armed And Really Pissed.)[39] Surging anti-AARP sentiment on the blogs and elsewhere registered with the burgeoning antigovernment Tea Party movement, which sponsored an AARP membership card–burning gathering in Washington, D.C., in early December.

FORMING COALITIONS IN UNSTABLE POLICY TERRAIN

In past, present, and future policy debates, AARP's leaders must negotiate difficult and shifting policy terrain with other powerful players. In building coalitions, by and large, Bill Novelli's AARP tried to maintain pragmatic, center-left positions. Divided We Fail was a pioneering coalition made up of the Business Roundtable, the National Federation of Independent Businesses, and the SEIU. Eventually, however, this very loose coalition showed strains: In his own considerable efforts at promoting health care reform, SEIU's savvy president Andy Stern rarely mentioned Divided We Fail or AARP; Stern and his union were more often identified with later alliances such as Better Health Care Together (with major corporate partners such as Walmart, General Mills, and AT&T) and with the Quality Care Coalition (which included the American Medical Association, Families USA, and the Federation of American Hospitals). The National Federation of Independent Businesses eventually urged its members to lobby Congress to vote against H.R. 3200.[40] AARP was also a coalition partner in Healthy Economy Now with the pharmaceutical lobby PhRMA and the Federation of American Hospitals, but this coalition dissolved when the other partners moved on to form Americans for Stable Quality Care.[41] On its own, however, AARP was successful in negotiating with the powerful pharmaceutical lobby for reduced drug prices for seniors in the Medicare "doughnut-hole" drug coverage gap.

On entitlement matters in general, AARP's leaders have negotiated with powerful policy players on the political right and the left. They dealt with the George W. Bush White House for eight years and continue dialogues with entitlement "fiscal hawks" in foundations, think tanks, the press, and Congress. The new Peter G. Peterson Foundation—with chief spokesman David Walker, former Congressional Budget Office director—has had considerable media impact. (Walker was a guest speaker at AARP's National Policy Agenda meetings in February 2008.)[42] The *Washington Post* columnist Robert Samuelson remains the foremost press critic of entitlement funding levels. Kent Conrad (D-SD) and Senator Judd Gregg (R-NH), among fiscal centrists in the Senate, and "Blue Dog Democrats" in the House will likely shape entitlement change.[43]

On the political left, a phalanx of more liberal unions, civil rights groups, and other interest groups had hopes for greater empowerment from a Democratic Congress and White House. The Obama administration's strong push for comprehensive health care reform heeded calls for more equitable universal health care by liberal groups such as the SEIU, the National Coalition for Healthcare Reform (led by the civil rights veteran Ralph Neas), and Families USA (helmed by its able lobbyist and founder Ron Pollack).[44] And AARP is the mighty anchor for a loose alliance of sixty other senior citizen service and advocacy groups, the Leadership Council of Aging Organizations.

In the realm of age-based politics, AARP remains without competitors. The conservative American Seniors' Association gained a few thousand AARP defectors during the health care reform battles, but it and other "conservative AARP alternatives" remain insignificant players. And instead of generational clashes with an Obama-energized youth movement, cooperation prevailed on health care reform between AARP and "Organizing for America," a revived and retooled version of the Internet-based campaign organization that elected Obama—initially referred to as "Obama 2.0." During the health care debates, Organizing for America sent messages to thirteen million e-mail addresses, four million cell phone contacts, and two million active volunteers. But its impact was negligible compared to the squads of angry senior citizens who turned out for August congressional town hall meetings.[45] (These developments distressed *New York Times* star editorial doyen Maureen Dowd: "Instead of a multicultural tableau of beaming young idealists on screen, we see ugly scenes of mostly older and white malcontents, disrupting forums where others have come to actually learn something. . . . Instead of hope, we get swastikas, death threats and T-shirts proclaiming 'Proud Member of the Mob.'")[46]

MISSION ACCOMPLISHED—AND REASSESSED

More than a decade after our first conversation about boomers in late 1999, John Rother, AARP's policy director and resident "boomer brain," had moved up from a more modest lower-floor office in AARP's massive headquarters building to a larger tenth-story office with an impressive view of the Capitol. He was generally pleased with the new PPACA and AARP's major role in achieving the milestone legislation.[47]

But Rother was disappointed by older Americans' sharply negative response to health care reform. AARP's own membership surveys found a somewhat less divided fifty-plus population. But the volume and visibility of intense, angry response registered on AARP's own Web page, elsewhere in the blogosphere, and in the contentious August town hall meetings was, Rother admitted, "extraordinary."

Those over sixty-five were the most vehemently opposed. But Rother was especially vexed by the lack of support from the age fifty to sixty-four baby boomer demographic. They were among the primary beneficiaries of the reform legislation's two major accomplishments: prohibiting the use of preexisting conditions to deny health insurance and setting limits on the use of age categories to determine insurance premiums.

Approximately four hundred thousand AARP members resigned in direct response to the organization's support of PPACA; perhaps another half million did not renew because of it. Rother figured it would take about a year to rebound via new member registration. Significantly, the losses were greatest among older, higher-income white men, a core constituency of and driving force behind the Tea Party movement.

The emergence of the boomer-driven Tea Party movement surprised Rother and others at ARRP. He took this as evidence of a broader reactionary or conservative response among aging boomers. Their more youthful protests against the status quo were yielding to fear of change, a response more typical of older adults.

Yet Rother remained more convinced than ever of boomers' basic ideological stability. "A generation's circumstances may change, but not their underlying mind-set." Aging boomers retained their characteristic individualism, desire for choices, and mistrust of government—the latter, perhaps, made even worse by the eight years of George W. Bush's administration. Not even the stock market crash, recession, and layoffs had changed that. Boomers' political potential has been lost—so far.

Nevertheless, Rother thought that many boomers were passing through a definitive life transition: the loss of their parents. Boomers increasingly must face the grim realization that *they* are the "older generation." Though many must still support their grown children (to a greater degree than their parents supported them), many are considering one final act of individual action and defiance: "reinvention." (AARP has taken note of this generational urge for a final metamorphosis via new television ads that teasingly begin: "When I grow up, I want to . . .")[48]

A fifty-year-old AARP is facing similar questions of organizational identity. Through 2009, AARP stayed the course on its long-term, expansive "big picture" strategy charted by Bill Novelli. They pursued the goal of preserving Medicare through broader health care reform, accepting the need for "efficiency" and cost control measures. AARP's leaders were probably correct in thinking that without overall health care reform Medicare would soon emerge as single, huge target for even more drastic cost cutting. Second, they were mindful that the organization could not win the membership and allegiance of future generations by ignoring the growing tax burdens imposed upon them by unreformed Medicare and Social Security systems. And, third, they realized that an inflexible defense of the entitlement status quo would reinforce AARP's "greedy geezer" stereotype.

By vigorously exercising its "warrior brand" in support of Democratic health care reform proposals, AARP risked compromising its commercial, nonpartisan trust brand so vital in marketing its "member value" products and services and in expanding its membership base. But in terms of membership or image, the organization escaped with little damage. Indeed, the campaign for health care reform and other issues, in combination with the general transformation of AARP under Bill Novelli, may have done much to reduce its "greedy geezer" stereotype—at least among AARP members. In a 2010 survey on civic engagement, only 16.7 percent of AARP members indicated that they belonged to an "organization for older people."[49]

AARP's leaders and research staff seem genuinely committed to fulfilling their "power to make it better" slogan through fostering more expansive "positive social change." They share the same general worries as America's corporate, educational, and political leaders about the growing economic gap between the "haves" and the "have-nots" across all generations. They are very much aware of the nation's changing demographics and ethnic composition. AARP pulses with the educated, upper-middle-class faith of the best and the brightest that economic and social problems can be managed with proper information, feedback, and measurement "metrics." They have been frustrated by the paralyzing political polarization in Washington, D.C., and the nation at large.

But the health care reform wars revealed within AARP two common sociological problems that tend to develop in large, established membership organizations. First, as the late Seymour Martin Lipset's classic study *Union Democracy* demonstrated, leadership can become ideologically insulated, aloof, and detached from its members' everyday concerns. Second, expanding, well-funded organizations may take on too many projects, resulting in loss of identity, loss of focus, and "mission drift." (As mentioned in chapter 5, there was muttering within AARP that the organization was becoming so broad based that it might be renamed "the American Association of Persons.")

Thus, while AARP's leadership cadre became more expansive and ambitious in reforming society and in representing "everyone who has a birthday," tens of thousands of its members felt that AARP had betrayed them by straying from what they considered its paramount political mission: protecting Medicare and Social Security. AARP's members over age sixty-five did not like the new face of a "power-to-make-it better" social change organization that appealed to aging boomers' 1960s social movement aspirations.[50] And, as discussed above, AARP's leaders were unprepared for the negative shift in senior sentiment toward comprehensive health care reform.

Ultimately, whether or not a significant number of AARP's members disapprove of its "nonpartisan" partisan politics, ideology and culture, one must credit the organization and its leaders for exercising much-needed leadership and long-term vision on one of the most vexing public policy issues of the twenty-first century. Few others did so. Divided We Fail offered a blueprint for change, and its basic elements were incorporated into the most significant piece of reform legislation since Medicare.

Furthermore, through their grassroots activism, AARP fostered necessary political awareness, discussion, and action that are the essence of democratic process and very much in the Ethel Percy Andrus tradition of "promoting positive change." AARP has become something of the "national forum" to discuss important issues that has been so longed for by the National Public Radio commentator Dick Meyer and many others. Though there may be an elite, left-leaning bias and though there may be some organizational financial interests at play, AARP's officers, board members, and researchers seem to be able to focus upon the national interest in a more nonpartisan manner than most other powerhouse policy players. But in a rapidly changing nation, the question is whether devotion to their founder's altruistic, happy mantra of "what we do, we do for all"—along with maintaining public trust in their products and financial services—ultimately compromises their "warrior brand" mission to advocate aggressively for older Americans' specific interests in possible opposition to the needs and desires of younger and middle-aged generations.

The Great Recession and the new era of limits have taken a toll on AARP's ambitions. In 2009, AARP suffered its worst financial setback in history, which resulted in layoffs of 10 percent of its staff and cutbacks in all major programs. (The organization advocating for careful retirement planning braved a measure of public ridicule by temporarily suspending its contributions to employee retirement accounts.)

Bill Novelli's ambitious global and multigenerational agendas have been scaled back. The new president, Barry Rand, reportedly wants the organization to become more focused and "member driven" and to try to create a "sense of community" for fifty-plus Americans. AARP's career fairs have drawn overflow crowds, and its massive Web page has been redesigned once again. A new "director of creative initiatives" has been hired.

AARP has expended much time and energy explaining and defending the new PPACA. These efforts will need to be redoubled in the wake of 2010 Republican congressional victories.

The ballooning national debt and sluggish economy now appear to be the crises so many experts deemed necessary to even consider serious entitlement reforms. Hence, AARP's "ultimate battle" is coming much closer: defending Medicare and Social Security through politically shaping policy changes.

Indeed, in December 2010, AARP had to confront a serious new salvo of entitlement reductions proposed by the National Commission on Fiscal Responsibility and Reform. The eighteen-member bipartisan panel had been appointed by President Obama and was cochaired by Erskine Bowles, former Clinton White House chief of staff, and by AARP's resolute Republican foe, the former U.S. Senator from Wyoming, Alan Simpson. A majority of the members approved the final report but it failed to attain the full endorsement of fourteen members—a required threshold for Congressional consideration of its recommendations. Yet the panel's package of tax reforms and entitlement reductions was surprisingly well received by pundits, politicians, and President Obama. But on AARP's web page, John Rother responded sharply to the commission's proposed changes in Social Security and Medicare. "The impact is troubling," Rother warned. The commission's proposals "would lower the retirement incomes of average people who rely on Social Security while significantly increasing their out of pocket costs for Medicare." In the January/February issue of the *AARP Bulletin*, CEO A. Barry Rand rattled his "warrior brand" sword, labeling the proposals as a "call to action for AARP. We're fighting to protect the retirement security of American families and future generations."

But whether aging boomers will follow AARP into battle remains an open question.

CHAPTER SEVEN

You Can't Always Get What You Want

Me, We, or AARP?

November 4, 2008, is a historic day because it marks the end
of an economic era, a political era and a generational era all
at once. Economically, it marks the end of the Long Boom
which began in 1983. Politically, it probably marks the end of
conservative dominance which began in 1980. Generationally,
it marks the end of baby boomer supremacy, which began
in 1968.

 —David Brooks (2008)

The biggest, but most underreported, financial story in
America is the looming retirement disaster. Eighty million
baby boomers are approaching retirement and most have
absolutely no idea what's going to hit them. For them the
financial crisis isn't over. It's just about to begin.

 —Brett Arends (2010)

Deep into the Great Recession summer of 2009, the career consultant
Carleen MacKay noticed that boomers' hallmark individualism and
optimism were sources of frustration: these traits blocked recognition and understanding of major systemic, economic changes. Aging
boomers attending her lectures or workshops retained a dogmatic
faith that if they tweaked resumes and made cosmetic changes (losing

weight, plastic surgery) their persistent individual efforts would yield "one more job" (secure and full time) like the one they had before—in occupational sectors that were, in fact, rapidly shrinking. "They're still looking for twentieth-century promises to be kept," said MacKay.[1]

Indeed, boomers' "Me Generation" heritage of individualism, confidence, and can-do optimism remained surprisingly strong during the Great Recession. A 2009 Focalyst survey found that only 25 percent of boomers were downbeat, backward-looking members of a "Yesterday" segment. Thirty percent fell into a "Today" segment that was fairly upbeat and of the opinion that "we live in exciting times." And a full 45 percent were classified in the "Tomorrow" segment, characterized by the belief that tomorrow would be better than today.[2] Most mainstream media coverage of the present and future retirement crises (as well as boomers' own postings on the Web and Internet) has emphasized individual solutions, not collective political action.

But deeper, darker currents of doubt and fear were also awakened. The real estate and stock market meltdowns and the consequent severe recession stirred Older Boomers' memories of their parents' stories of widespread hardship during the Great Depression. Peggy Noonan observed that "those thinking about retirement are just old enough to remember America before the abundance, before everyone was rich, rich being defined as plenty to eat, a stable place to live and some left over for fun and pleasure. For them, the crash has released old memories. And it's spooking people."[3]

"We're seeing values and behaviors going back to the Depression," declared Jody Holtzman, AARP's senior vice president for thought leadership, whose research staff had just conducted a survey of consumer attitudes and behavior of Americans over forty-five. "It's cash only, they're saving and they're going out less."[4]

Older Boomers (born 1946–55) are becoming a culturally conscious generation, but they are not yet a politically conscious one.[5] They are growing comfortable with the term and identity of "boomer" because they are linked together by common history and memories, made manifest in nostalgia for the popular culture of their youth—especially rock music and television. Animated by these new cultural forces in the 1960s, youthful college-educated boomers protested inequities in "the System" and set in motion many important cultural and institutional changes, especially in reducing discrimination against minorities, women, and gays and lesbians. Many boomers were instrumental in the "change we can believe in" presidential campaign of Barack Obama and are active in his administration.

In the aftermath of bursting residential real estate bubbles, the stock market meltdown and the Great Recession, many aging boomers are economically anxious, unquestionably more aware of their shared economic and retirement vulnerabilities. And AARP has been reminding boomers of their advancing age and retirement anxieties through its stepped-up advertising and its famous saturation mass-mailing campaigns.

The predisposing sociological factors for the emergence of generational mobilization and protest would seem to be perfectly aligned: rising economic tensions, structural strain, political polarization, a growing sense of crisis, and precipitating events, such as a deep recession, layoffs, and the looming fight over Medicare and Social Security changes. Yet the most striking finding about boomers' senior power potential is its absence—so far. Why?

Carleen MacKay concluded that mounting job losses were not yet sufficiently threatening to galvanize collective action. "It is not at the point yet where enough people (boomers) have been impacted directly so terribly that they're willing to take a stance—yet."[6] This has been true especially for the approximately one-third of Older Boomers who have college degrees. As discussed in chapter 4, the 2010 Metlife report on the Great Recession's impact on Older Boomers indicates that those with college degrees have better prospects for maintaining their jobs and salaries than do than their non-college-educated generational brethren.[7] The Great Recession has adversely affected far more Americans in the managerial and professional classes than did previous economic downturns; but these upscale, unemployed casualties have not responded collectively or politically.[8] Again, why?

Carleen MacKay observed that boomers experiencing job or career setbacks often expressed disenchantment with government—but also feelings of personal alienation, powerlessness, and passivity. "People feel so disenfranchised they don't know how to *act*. They feel defeated, and [they feel,] 'There's not much I can do about it anyway, so better hunker down and take care of myself.'"[9] These sentiments hardly constitute the high-octane fuel required for a robust generational voting bloc or political protest movement.

As emphasized in chapter 3, aging boomers' continuing ideological emphases upon individual responsibility, self-blame, and do-it-yourself solutions block communication about common problems, the necessary precursor to generating a sense of urgency, moral outrage, and a widespread feeling that "something needs to be done." These factors, in turn, are essential in spurring political mobilization and proposals for systemic reform. Additionally, instead of rising generational economic and sociological convergence, deepening class and educational gaps sharply divide boomers against themselves politically and culturally. Boomer elites and professional classes embrace supercapitalism, globalization, multiculturalism, progressive politics, and social engineering, while more vulnerable middle- and working-class boomers fear or mistrust those forces.[10] Class-based cultural divides, do-it-yourself individualism, and negative boomer stereotypes—often generated by boomers themselves—remain the most formidable obstacles to any sort of age-based voting bloc or movement mobilization to defend Social Security, Medicare, or other entitlements.

WHEN THERE'S NO "ONE MORE TOMORROW"

If there is not another period of prolonged prosperity and/or a steady rise in stock market values during the next decade, a majority of Older

Boomers will be as dependent upon Medicare and Social Security as their parents were. As suggested in chapter 4, there are preliminary signs that even antigovernment Tea Party boomers are becoming aware of this dilemma.[11]

But mere talk of entitlement reductions thus far has not mobilized larger numbers of boomers because most are still employed. Despite stock market and real estate declines coupled with rising unemployment or the fear of it, most Older Boomers still assume that there is more time, "one more tomorrow." But in five or ten years, there will be no more "tomorrows" in terms of retirement planning.

Thus there is the potential catalyst of "the crisis next time," a slow-growth economy coupled with a future financial panic or entitlement crisis that would hit millions of Older Boomers when they are fully retired, unable to continue or resume working, and dependent upon retirement accounts, Social Security, and Medicare. Direct, immediate experience of Social Security or Medicare cutbacks by retired boomers might finally elicit a mass political response. ("When my Social Security check is actually cut in half, that's when I'll get mad," *Examiner.com* baby boomer columnist Paul Briand informed me.)[12]

Generational leadership might also galvanize aging boomers' identity, raise consciousness, and inspire collective political action. But there is no self-identified champion of aging boomers' interests.

I asked nearly everyone interviewed for this book: Who speaks for boomers? Who might be their leader, their Claude Pepper (the late U.S. senator from Florida, long identified as the Senate's champion for senior citizens)? Virtually everyone answered, in so many words, "No one I can think of." Practically no one suggested AARP.

Yet AARP is the only organization capable of framing, debating, and mobilizing a defense of entitlements and other issues of concern to older Americans. In the absence of a new Claude Pepper or any collective "we" in the form of a voting bloc or broadly-based boomer political movement, AARP remains the de facto political voice for aging Americans. But AARP's commitment to Medicare and Social Security is now questioned by millions of boomers and older Americans who suspect that AARP sold them out by supporting real or alleged rationing and redistribution embodied in the newly enacted Patient Protection and Affordable Care Act. AARP will probably survive this crisis, as it has others in the past. Lately, the organization is earning considerable goodwill by sponsoring forty-eight job fairs for older Americans in nineteen states. As its critics complain, AARP is "too big to fail."

But whither the nation-state in an era of globalization and declining levels of interpersonal and institutional trust?

ONE NATION: DIVIDED AND UNCERTAIN

Aging boomers and AARP will continue their political mating dance in a rapidly changing society. One reason the health care reform debates became so polarizing was that they were connected to unasked, highly sensitive questions involving the impact of supercapitalism, immigration, and globalization upon national identity, interpersonal and institutional trust, and the future of the nation-state and the civic solidarity that underpins Social Security, Medicare, and the spirit of *E Pluribus Unum*.

Today, as Robert Reich has emphasized, global supercapitalism has sapped the cooperative spirit of the social compact, civic society, and *E Pluribus Unum* by making an international bounty of market choices available to individual consumers and investors.[13] And as Robert Putnam's politically inconvenient survey research findings demonstrate, increasing ethnic diversity erodes the "social networks and associated norms of reciprocity and trustworthiness" that hold civic society together.[14] Yet these processes and consequences are only dimly seen or are simply denied by the nation's leaders.

One of the most amazing discoveries of my years of field research and conversations with experts on the subject of aging baby boomers was that practically no one had considered the "big picture" question of how to maintain mid-twentieth-century nation-state entitlements in the midst of twenty-first-century change. Social Security and Medicare were seen as problematic; so were political polarization and declining levels of trust in government; but the rapidly changing demographic and institutional contexts were not considered at all.

When I did raise these questions, nearly all those I talked with were initially intrigued, even excited—until and unless the tabooed subject of immigration was mentioned. Then, in many situations, the atmosphere grew somewhat anxious or defensive. Sometimes the topic of immigration was dismissed as unimportant or as a diversion promoted by talk-radio or former CNN pundit Lou Dobbs. Officially, AARP has been mute on the subject: immigration as a political or public policy issue is not discussed in its publications—though cultural diversity is studied and celebrated.[15]

The deep perceptual divisions between the nation's elites and America's middle and working classes on the consequences of global supercapitalism and immigration augur similar conflicts on entitlement reform. As seen in previous chapters, immigration has been the unacknowledged "elephant in the room" in public debates about health care, Social Security, and Medicare reform.[16]

California's immigration-driven, age/ethnic/class divisions are spreading into much of metropolitan America.[17] This increasingly alarms corporate, government, and public policy leaders attuned to the health of the nation's civic and volunteer organizations. Several organizations and foundations (including the U.S. government's Corporation for National and Community Service, AARP, and the well-known nonprofit group Civic Ventures) have launched major initiatives to foster volunteerism and civic engagement—with a special eye toward recruiting millions of retired baby boomers.[18]

Advocates of civic engagement campaigns and entitlement reform have assumed that boomers will want to "give back" to society and leave a positive legacy because they have cherished children and grandchildren. ("Preserving Social Security for future generations" is now an

AARP mantra.) And many polls indicate boomers' desire to engage in volunteer or civic efforts.

Yet the Yankelovich researchers J. Walker Smith and Ann Clurman warned that boomers have little interest in a long-term "legacy" except in terms of how well they defend their own interests in the here and now. "Boomers want a mission, but not to leave a legacy. They want to make a difference for themselves today."[19] As for volunteerism, self-interested boomers have a preference for quick, specialized relationships (enhanced by modern technologies) that may produce transitory "connections without community," not the broad, diffuse bonds required for social capital.[20] (In January 2009, AARP confirmed such insights by launching its "Create the Good" Web site so that members with limited time could quickly access online forums and search databases for civic involvement opportunities.)

The stock market dive and Great Recession have led to sobering reassessments as to how many boomers might be able or willing to participate in civic renewal. One Beltway proponent of these initiatives told me:

> This [boomer] generation has had a unique combination of leisure, wealth, and some kind of civic orientation. Perfect ingredients! But what is the impact of this current financial crisis? One-third of that retirement wealth that created the space for people to do all this stuff has disappeared. And work-life needs to be extended [and] may crowd out all that. There's this weird feeling that we were dealing with something of a bubble of civic possibility and it was rising and suddenly it just lost all the air—before it really happened. It was just coming together. This is a huge challenge to us.[21]

By 2010, an AARP survey entitled "Connecting and Giving" emphasized that midlife and older Americans were less optimistic about the potential of civic activities and were more individually and sporadically involved than in the past. "The fragmentation of American life," wrote the report's authors, "is a challenge for membership organizations . . . that rely on formal, volunteer support."[22] The impact of the economic meltdown on the nation's educated upper middle classes confirmed critics' suspicions that the well-publicized civic engagement crusade was tacitly geared to relatively well-off, educated Americans (or those with generous pensions) who had the leisure time and resources to volunteer.

Even if economic conditions improve, mobilizing aging boomers for civic renewal may be as difficult as generating political consciousness and action. As discussed in chapters 1 and 2, it is important to remember that approximately one-third of boomers have only one child or are childless; others may be alienated from their children because of divorce, geographical distance, or other factors. (Even within their own families, aging boomers are being forced to choose between investing for retirement or putting aside funds for their children's college education. The *Wall Street Journal* columnist Jeff Opdyke and his spouse pondered this choice and decided: "I think that instead of a free ride through college, a better gift to my kids is a mom and dad financially self-sufficient in their dotage.")[23]

In a world of global supercapitalism, mass migrations, and eroding trust and national identity, the coming debates over old-age entitlements raise fundamental questions about the nature of the social order, social cohesion, and the durability of the social contract between generations, between employers and employees, and between state and citizens: What is a nation? What do we owe one another? Who are we? What holds us together? Is there a shared vision of the future?

Change, dissolution, and decline are old themes in the social sciences. In the nineteenth century the massive social upheavals caused by the Twin Revolutions (Industrial and French) led to the founding of sociology, the field that focuses on sources and impact of social order, social cohesion, and social change. France's Alexis de Tocqueville, August Comte, and Emile Durkheim, and Germany's Karl Marx, Ferdinand Tonnies, and Max Weber, focused on the impact of industrialization and spreading democracy on the key institutions of community, tradition, authority, religion, social class, moral order, and shared values.[24]

At the end of the nineteenth century, Oswald Spengler mourned "the decline of the West."

Likewise, political elites' worries about class polarization and declining social cohesion date at least as far back as ancient Rome. In terms of U.S. history, the most direct parallel to the current century is the dawn of the previous one. Theodore Roosevelt and the founders of the Progressive movement were deeply concerned about alleviating problems posed by industrialization, mass immigration, and class polarization. The Progressive era gave birth to today's faith that changing and managing the social environment could change human behavior. The many reforms of the Progressive era from 1900 to 1920 were designed to blunt class conflict, institutionalize labor-management negotiations, "Americanize" immigrants, and quench the appeal of anarchist and socialist solutions. The redistributive reforms of Franklin Roosevelt's New Deal in the 1930s served similar ends. Social Security was founded during a time of intensely felt national crisis, and thirty years later Medicare was born in the consensus, hope, and optimism of the 1960s Great Society.

Today, the industrial nation-state that gave birth to the boomers and to old-age entitlements is morphing into something else. We are not yet sure what this "New America" (as Peggy Noonan terms it) will look like. We do receive daily reminders of the passing of the "Old America." Two of the most poignant were the deaths of former CBS news anchor Walter Cronkite and Senator Ted Kennedy in 2009. In the 1960s and 1970s, Cronkite had symbolized something of a one-man national consensus, a unifying, reassuring, trusted source who seemed to transcend societal differences. Asked by MSNBC's Rachel Maddow if there could ever again be such a figure in American news media, the current NBC Evening News anchor Brian Williams quickly responded, "No. We're too fragmented now."[25] And Senator Ted Kennedy was the embodiment of the Old America's can-do spirit and optimistic trust in big-government programs. No more.

THE TRUST BUST

Within weeks of Senator Kennedy's death, as the political sound and fury escalated about proposed congressional health care reforms, Andrew Kohut, president of the Pew Research Center, pondered whether the original 1965 Medicare legislation might today be met with the same doubt, skepticism, and polarization. He concluded it would. The reason: "Broad distrust of government—which was not evident in the 1960s—is an important reason why Americans are reacting so differently to health care reform in 2009 than they did in 1965." In the late 1950s, Kohut discovered, 65 percent of Americans trusted the national government to do the right thing always or most of the time. By 1974, only 36 percent did. And the trust in government has never been recovered.[26]

The policy scholar Elaine Kamarck warned excited fellow Democrats about the "Trust Challenge" in a 2008 paper entitled "Change You Can Believe In Needs a Government You Can Trust."[27] Like Kohut, Kamarck marshaled polling data to demonstrate fifty years of declining public trust that that government would do the right thing "just about always or most of the time." She argued that declining trust in government had produced the "postbureaucratic state," in which new policies moved away from direct taxation or regulation and increasingly toward substituting market-based incentives (such as those used in the federal regulation of sulfur dioxide and in the proposed "cap and trade" system for carbon dioxide controls). And policy implementation was increasingly carried out by public/private hybrid organizations (via subcontracting and outsourcing) rather than by government agencies. After the autumn of 2008, however, Kamarck found that professional and public trust in market-driven systems had collapsed along with the stock market.[28]

"Will We Ever Trust Wall Street Again?" asked veteran *Wall Street Journal* columnist Jason Zweig, who observed that the financial crisis severely threatened average investors' beliefs in a "just world" of free markets, individual responsibility, and investing for the future.[29] Former Federal Reserve chair Paul Volcker sensed rising popular mistrust of business and government collusion. "It's good to be skeptical about government. We ought to be skeptical. But at the bottom, you know, we need some trust that these officials are there, they're responsible, they're doing the best they can in the interest of the country. A lot of that's been lost, [there's] this feeling that the lobbyists are controlling everything and the amount of money involved is enormous, which it is."[30] The Republican pollster Frank Luntz added his concern: "For business and political elites, the message is clear: Restore trust."[31]

By 2010 a Pew Research Center report revealed "a perfect storm of conditions associated with distrust of government: a dismal economy, an unhappy public, bitter partisan-based backlash, and epic discontent with Congress and elected officials." Age was not a major variable, but political affiliation was: nearly 80 percent of all age groups—with the exception of 67 percent of adults under thirty—thought government could be trusted to do what was right only some of the time or never. Eighty-six percent of Republicans agreed, as did 79 percent of Independents, but only 64 percent of Democrats. Ninety-two percent of those who approved of the Tea Party movement also agreed. (Nearly two-thirds of respondents held negative views of banks, other financial institutions, and large corporations, while majorities darkly regarded the national news media and the entertainment industry; 49 percent had negative views of labor unions, while only 32 percent held positive views.)[32]

Many liberals had hoped that the 2008 election of Barack Obama and a Democratic Congress would bring the return of something like the New Deal. (A postelection *Time* magazine cover portrayed Obama as Franklin Roosevelt complete with top hat and cigarette holder.) Indeed, despite the rising tide of public mistrust of government, the most progressive legislative landmarks in decades have been enacted: the Patient Protection and Affordable Care Act (PPACA) and the

Dodd–Frank Wall Street Reform and Consumer Protection Act. Yet these reforms seem to lack widespread public understanding and support. The 2010 Republican congressional victories threaten to stall or compromise this new legislation through funding cutbacks or changes or delays in implementation.

As pointed out in previous chapters, boomers have been fragmented in their responses to both the economic crises and increasing threats to Social Security and Medicare. Baby boomers have been among the leaders in both Obama's presidential campaign and the Tea Party movement. But will any political party or organization—specifically AARP—be able to win the allegiance of a "critical mass" of rank-and-file boomers, especially the Older Boomers who are just now beginning to assume a sense of "ownership" of Social Security and Medicare? Who will win the boomers' trust? Or will masses of boomer individuals ultimately trust only in themselves?

ME, WE, OR AARP?

I shall end this book with the question posed at the beginning: Will aging boomers become an awakening, age-conscious political giant, increasingly visible either as an inert voting bloc or as a more active political movement geared to the protection of Medicare and Social Security? Can aging boomers transcend their many internal cultural, economic, and political differences and vote their age-based interests, fulfilling the presumption of age-motivated voting in the "senior power model" challenged by Robert Binstock? And what will be the role of AARP?

Boomers' senior power potential will be heavily influenced by the nation's economic future. Another decade of stagnant stock and real estate markets coupled with a long "jobless recovery" will increase aging boomers' collective sense of angst and vulnerability—but also entangle Social Security and Medicare funding battles with rising economic and social problems of other population segments, especially in the wake of the Great Recession. In a widely read *Atlantic* magazine cover story, senior editor Don Peck listed these problems: "A slowly sinking [younger] generation; a remorseless assault on the identity of many men; the dissolution of families and the collapse of neighborhoods; a thinning veneer of national amity—the social legacies of the Great Recession are still being written, but their breadth and depth are immense. As problems, they are enormously complex and their solutions will be equally so."[33] How will these forces shape boomers' political choices of "Me, We, or AARP"?

Should boomers remain fragmented by class, educational, cultural, and other differences, then the "politics of me" will prevail, an individualized, issue-oriented politics of "tailored engagement" predicted in the 2004 AARP study *A Changing Political Landscape*. Instead of a rerun of 1960s mass protests, aging boomer politics will be narrowly issue oriented, reflecting a more limited political involvement style, operating outside the traditional two-party system via Web-based communities and "checkbook activism."[34] Boomers' "strong sense of entitlement and self-directed motivations will help to create a more decentralized, broader, community-based path for activism."[35]

A "politics of we," a boomer-based voting bloc or political movement, could still emerge in response to aggressive White House and congressional efforts to reduce Social Security benefits or to ration Medicare directly or indirectly. The five-hundred-billion-dollar cut in projected increases in Medicare spending contained in the 2010 PPACA has already energized groups of boomers and seniors and led to Republican pledges to "repeal" PPACA after the 2010 elections. The Great Recession has raised Older Boomers' preretirement anxieties and vulnerabilities: a majority are now more clearly aware that they are financially unprepared for retirement. This is likely one reason why age joined the key variables of class and race in structuring voting behavior in the 2008 presidential election, especially in the Democratic primary contest between Barack Obama and Hillary Clinton.

A third, middle-ground, cooperative scenario may well emerge through AARP's de facto leadership in defining and brokering aging boomers' health care and retirement interests with the rest of American society. In spite of its controversial, partisan support of the Democrats' successful comprehensive health care reform, the "nonpartisan" organization endures as one of the nation's most trusted institutions. Through its outreach to younger generations and its keen awareness of the changing demographic makeup of the nation, AARP has positioned itself as the arbiter of generational equity and the champion of the social contract that underpins Medicare and Social Security.

AARP's increasing emphasis on intergenerational cooperation and equity is being echoed by popular pundits on both the left and the right. The liberal *New York Times* columnist Thomas Friedman advocates "regeneration," emphasizing that "we have to pay for more new schools and infrastructure than ever, while accepting more entitlement cuts than ever, when public trust in government is lower than ever."[36] His conservative *Times* colleague David Brooks has called for a "Geezer Crusade," recognizing that "only the old can lead a generativity revolution—millions of people demanding changes in health care spending and the retirement age to make life better for their grandchildren."[37]

But happy talk of intergenerational generosity may be a tough sell. Brooks's proposal for a Geezer Crusade was greeted with scorn by many online responders, including one "reader-recommended" commenter, a likely boomer cynic, who jeered, "Dream on, Dude."

Calls for generational confrontation have also appeared in the *Times:* "Are We Overpaying Grandpa?" the University of Chicago economist Casey Mulligan pointedly asked. She noted that the elderly receive a disproportionate amount of government spending, an average $40,000 each. Combined with their private incomes and home-based wealth, their living standard far exceeds that of the average American. Mulligan posed a blunt challenge. "The question for the future of Medicare is this: Are families ready to triple their spending on the health care of their highest-income family members?"[38]

THE STAGE IS SET: THE FIGHT BEGINS

The entitlement time bomb is ticking. Changes are inevitable. In 2010, for the first time, working Americans' annual Social Security Statement carried the following warning on its front page:

About Social Security's Future

Social Security is a compact between generations. Since 1935, America has kept the promise of security for its workers and their families. Now, however, the Social Security system is facing serious financial problems, and action is needed soon to make sure the system will be sound when today's younger workers are readying for retirement.

In 2016 we will begin paying more in benefits than we collect in taxes. Without changes, by 2037 the Social Security Trust Fund will be exhausted and there will be enough money to pay only about 76 cents for each dollar of scheduled benefits. We need to resolve these issues soon to make sure Social Security continues to provide a foundation of protection for future generations.

In 1990, Medicare and Social Security represented 28 percent of federal spending; by 2019, that figure may approach 40 percent. The nation's economic future is uncertain—as are the sociological cohesion and intergenerational solidarity of the Western world's aging nation-states. Indeed, in Greece and in France, recent entitlement changes provoked strikes and civil unrest. Most probably that will not happen here. Reforms of Social Security and Medicare will more likely entail prolonged political combat among pundits, policy makers, and think tanks, throughout Washington's vast lobbying labyrinth, and, ultimately, upon the battlefields in Congress—heavily influenced by the White House. All of them will be attuned to public opinion.

Americans appear about evenly divided on raising the eligibility ages for both Medicare and Social Security.[39] As for implementing private accounts for Social Security, a 2010 Pew Research Center study found that among respondents aged eighteen to twenty-nine, 70 percent were in favor of the idea versus 14 percent opposed; among those aged thirty to forty-nine, 63 percent were in favor, 23 percent opposed; among those aged fifty to sixty-four (baby boomers), 54 percent were in favor, 36 percent opposed; while among those aged sixty-five and over, 42 percent were in favor and 42 percent opposed.[40]

But the Pew Center study found that most age groups opposed replacing Medicare with an individualized voucher system: among those aged sixty-five and over, 69 percent were opposed versus 14 percent in favor; among those aged fifty to sixty-four, 57 percent were opposed versus 25 percent in favor; among those aged eighteen to twenty-nine, 53 percent were opposed versus 38 percent in favor; only those among those aged thirty to forty-nine were a majority in favor (48 percent, versus 37 percent opposed).

By the end of 2010, trial balloons for entitlement reforms were being lofted as a rising number of major pundits and policy makers proposed that the greater good of national debt reduction might justify Social Security and Medicare modifications. Major newspaper editorial pages and columnists began chipping away at Social Security's sacred status.[41]

In a popular *Time* magazine cover story, "Restoring the American Dream," the influential journalist Fareed Zakaria advanced a seductive growth-versus-entitlements argument that will be echoed in months to come. Zakaria prescribed vastly increased private investment and innovation and reduced consumption—the latter achieved, in part, through "radical rebalancing of government." This, in turn, would entail sharp reductions in health care and public pension spending— cuts that would hugely and disproportionately affect aging boomers.[42] Major think tank scholars have broached similar proposals for reducing the national debt through entitlement reforms.[43]

As noted in chapters 5 and 6, AARP has signaled that it is open to some degree of long-term change on Social Security and Medicare.[44] And, as mentioned at the close of the previous chapter, in late 2010 the National Commission on Fiscal Responsibility and Reform proposed entitlement reductions that were favorably received.

Without AARP's leadership and vast resources, aging boomers' abilities to politically resist entitlement reductions against progrowth appeals to "restore the middle class" and "reduce debt for our children" would be difficult at best. As argued in chapters 3 and 4, their willingness to mobilize on their own as a voting bloc or movement may be fatally compromised by long-standing class/political/cultural divides, negative self-publicity wrought by boomers bashing boomers, and increasing calls for generational sacrifice and atonement.[45]

On the other hand, the results of the 2010 elections probably raised levels of political polarization and stalemate in the nation (and, especially, in Washington, D.C.) to such a degree that no individual or party will dare offer—much less, successfully enact—major entitlement reforms until after the 2012 presidential elections.

But the stage is being set for entitlement reform. The fight over Social Security, Medicare, and the future of the American nation-state has begun. Divided or united, boomers will be in the thick of those battles. And, whether as advocate or mediator, so will AARP.

METHODOLOGICAL ODYSSEY

From Lonely Quest to a Bounty of Data

One Nation under AARP began about eleven years ago as a somewhat lonely and largely investigative, qualitative study that was gradually supplemented by an increasing amount of quantitative data gathered by others. The key question that informed the study was: How will aging baby boomers cope with getting older in a changing society? In what ways will their aging be similar to—or different from—that of previous generations? And, finally, if threatened cutbacks to pensions, Social Security, or Medicare emerged, would aging boomers politically mobilize to defend embattled entitlements?

A related—and originally very much hypothetical—question was posed in a 1997 PBS *Frontline* documentary, "Betting on the Market," that I still use in my undergraduate class "Inequality, Politics, and Public Policy." Long before Jacob Hacker wrote *Risk Shift*, this documentary illustrated the increasing dependence of baby boomers upon the stock market in financing their retirements. Though produced during the heady stock market boom of the 1990s, at the conclusion of the report its producer and narrator, Ron Chernow, paused to ponder: "What would happen if we had a sustained bear market after a lot of the baby boomers had retired? They were all past fifty-nine. They were beginning to draw from these different retirement plans that were invested in the stock market and yet, suddenly, their stocks were under water. On paper, their investments were down 30, 40, 50 percent. What would they do?"

I had no idea that there would be a sneak preview of Chernow's stock market meltdown scenario just I was trying to bring my research to a close in 2008.

A decade ago, I was amazed to find few other social scientists interested in the topic of aging boomers' politics and sociological future. The few books with "boomers" in the title went largely unsold and unnoticed. Some economists—many of the "doomsday" variety—were issuing grim projections on Social Security and Medicare. But in political science and sociology there was almost no interest. Nor were savvy Beltway political strategists aware of the impending clash of seventy-eight million baby boomers, a major recession, and strained and soon-to-be embattled entitlements.

The early and middle phases of the study, therefore, were much informed by "elite interviewing," interviews and conversations with some sixty persons in strategic organizational positions and with expertise on aging boomers in the areas of Medicare, social security, gerontology, and workforce issues. These included persons at the National Academy on an Aging Society, the Urban Institute, Brookings Institution, the Employee Benefits Research Institute, the U.S. Corporation for National Community Service, several anonymous sources in the U.S. Congress and the George W. Bush White House, the Alliance for Healthcare Reform, the National Committee for the Preservation of Social Security and Medicare, Merrill Lynch, Inc., Metlife Mature Market Institute, Eons.com, BBHQ.com, ThirdAge. com, and many other organizations. Over the years, through "snow-ball sampling," I worked my way to another twenty additional consultants, experts, and others interested in aging boomers—including some of the "frontline" career planners. [The general methodology of this research has been guided by two social science classics: Lewis Dexter, *Elite and Specialized Interviewing* (Northwestern University

Press, 1969) and Jack Douglas, *Investigative Social Research* (Sage Publications, 1976), as well as a more recent manual by Joseph A. Maxwell entitled *Qualitative Research Design: An Interactive Approach* (Sage Publications, 1996).]

Especially during the past two years, in the wake of the 2008 stock market crash and the onset of the Great Recession, it has become hard to keep count of all the people I've talked with about aging baby boomers, especially with regard to the numerous "reinterviews" and ongoing conversations I have repeatedly conducted over the years with a core group of experts and friends in a variety of settings. (The annual meetings of the American Society on Aging/National Conference on Aging have been fertile fields of data and insights.) Most people indulged me, knowing that Fred Lynch would inevitably start asking about and talking about "aging boomers" for the book he was forever writing.

The tempo and complexity of this research increased considerably in 2009 as the debate over comprehensive health care reform (and Medicare) began to emerge. Happily, this focused public and professional attention on many of my core topics, especially baby boomers and AARP. The long drought of secondary data turned into a flood of new data and reports on baby boomers—especially after the 2008 economic meltdowns. As a result, to some extent, the book has become not only a sociological field study but also a work on rapidly changing contemporary history.

The emerging central focus upon AARP in the book and its title grew out of my realization, during the research process, that "all roads led to AARP." They had—and still have—most of the data and expertise on aging baby boomers. It is still true, as I have often said, that "Nobody knows boomers like AARP." They are also well prepared for the coming debates over Social Security and Medicare. As I conclude in the book, currently there is simply no other organization that can lead, mobilize the troops, and fight the good fight to preserve these programs.

I especially wish to acknowledge the extensive time, accessibility, cordiality, cooperation, and insights of numerous AARP officers, editors, and research staff. They are indeed "Boomer Central." The surveys and focus group research conducted by their Public Policy Institute and Knowledge Management Division are extensively referenced throughout this book.

NOTES

INTRODUCTION

The Michael Moore chapter epigraph is from the interview with him in *Rolling Stone,* May 3–12, 2007.

1. See Robert Rich, *Supercapitalism* (New York: Alfred A. Knopf, 2008), and Fareed Zakaria, *The Post-American World* (New York: Norton, 2008).

2. "The New Global Elite," *Newsweek,* December 29, 2008.

3. John Zogby, *The Way We'll Be* (New York: Random House, 2008), 93.

4. The question of national social cohesion in Canada—and the split between the well-educated classes and the rest of the population—has been raised by the Liberal Party leader of the Canadian parliament, Michael Ignatieff, in his book *True Patriot Love: Four Generations in Search of Canada* (Toronto: Viking Canada, 2009).

5. Dick Meyer, *Why We Hate Us: American Discontent in a New Millennium* (New York: Crown, 2008), 209.

6. Judith Warner, "I Feel It Coming Together," *New York Times,* October 15, 2009.

7. Barbara Gordon, "Who Will Be 'Me' for Me?" *My Generation,* August 2002.

8. CNN Exit Poll, November 5, 2008, www.cnn.com/ELECTION/2008/results/polls/#USP00p1.

9. Ken Dychtwald, *Age Power: How the 21st Century Will Be Ruled by the New Old* (New York: Tarcher/Putnam, 1999).

10. Daniel Okrent, "Twilight of the Boomers," *Time,* June 12, 2000.

11. See Peter G. Peterson, *Running on Empty: How the Democratic and Republican Parties Are Bankrupting Our Future and What Americans Can Do about It* (New York: Farrar, Straus and Giroux, 2004), and *Gray Dawn: How the Coming Age Wave Will Transform America—and the World* (New York: Times Books/Random House, 1999).

12. See Ralph Turner and Lewis Killian, *Collective Behavior,* 3rd ed. (Englewood Cliffs, NJ: Prentice-Hall, 1987), 17–23.

13. See Alicia H. Munnell, Anthony Webb, and Luke Delorme, *A New National Retirement Risk Index,* Issue in Brief, no. 48 (Boston: Boston College Center for Retirement Research, June 2006); Alicia H. Munnell, Mauricio Soto, Anthony Webb, Francesca Golub-Sass, and Dan Muldoon, *Health Care Costs Drive Up the National Retirement Risk Index,* Issue in Brief, no. 8–3 (Boston: Boston College Center for Retirement Research, February 2008).

14. See Gary T. Marx and Douglas McAdam, *Collective Behavior and Social Movements: Process and Structure* (Englewood Cliffs, NJ: Prentice-Hall, 1994).

15. Tom Brokaw, *Boom! Voices of the Sixties* (New York: Random House, 2007), 578.

16. Michael Kinsley, "The Least We Can Do," *Atlantic Monthly,* October 2010.

17. George Anders, interview with the author, Claremont, CA, November 12, 1998.

18. Peterson, *Gray Dawn* and *Running on Empty;* Laurence J. Kotlikoff and Scott Burns, *The Coming Generational Storm: What You Need to Know about America's Economic Future* (Cambridge, MA: MIT Press, 2004); Alice M. Rivlin and Joseph R. Antos, eds., *Restoring Fiscal Sanity: The Health Spending Challenge* (Washington, DC: Brookings Institution Press, 2007); James Schulz and Robert Binstock, *Aging Nation: The Economics and Politics of Growing Older in America* (Westport, CT: Praeger, 2006); and Andrew L. Yarrow's *Forgive Us Our Debts: The Intergenerational Dangers of Fiscal Irresponsibility* (New Haven: Yale University Press, 2008).

19. Dana Milbank, "Smile—You're on Social Security!" *Washington Post,* October 16, 2007, A2.

20. Jacob Hacker, *The Great Risk Shift* (New York: Oxford University Press, 2006).

21. Quoted in Anne Tergesen, "How to Fix 401(k)s," *Wall Street Journal,* December 12, 2008.

22. On the basis of his substantial survey research data, the Harvard political scientist Robert Putnam reluctantly concluded that immigration-driven ethnic diversity weakens interpersonal trust and the web of friendships and associations that are the glue of civic society. See Robert D. Putnam, "*E Pluribus Unum:* Diversity and Community in the Twenty-first Century: The 2006 Johan Skytte Prize Lecture," *Scandinavian Political Studies* 30, no. 2 (2007): 151.

23. Ibid.

24. See William H. Frey, "America's Regional Demographics in the Early 21st Century: The Role of Seniors, Boomers and New Minorities," *Public Policy and Aging Report* 18 (Winter 2008): 1–31.

25. Peter Schrag, *California: America's High-Stakes Experiment* (Berkeley: University of California Press, 2006).

26. Dowell Myers, *Immigrants and Boomers: Forging a New Social Contract for the Future of America* (New York: Russell Sage Foundation, 2007); Michael Lind, "A Citizen-Based Social Contract," New America Foundation, Washington, DC, July 2007, www.newamerica.net/files/NSC%20Citizen%20Principles%20Paper%207–10–07.pdf; Mark Schmitt, "The American Social Contract: From Drift to Mastery," New America Foundation, Washington, DC, November 2007, www.newamerica.net/publications/policy/american_social_contract_drift_mastery; Cliff Zukin, "The American Public and the Next Social Contract," New America Foundation, Washington, DC, February 2008, http://newamerica.net/publications/policy/american_public_and_next_social_contract.

27. See Alan Berube et al., *State of Metropolitan America: On the Front Lines of Demographic Transformation* (Washington, DC: Brookings Institution, 2010).

1. BOOMER BASICS

The chapter epigraph is from Howard J. Fineman, "The Last Hurrah," *Newsweek,* January 23, 2006.

1. Mary S. Furlong, *Turning Silver into Gold* (Upper Saddle River, NJ: Financial Times Press, 2007).

2. For a somewhat similar account of a more recent conference on boomers as business opportunity, see Michael Winerip, "The Fountain of Reinvention," *New York Times,* April 22, 2010.

3. Jennifer Mann, "Baby Boomers Become the Forgotten Consumer," *Kansas City Star,* August 4, 2008. One year later, the marketing psychologist Paco Underhill offered the same lament: "Sixty percent of discretionary income

is in the hands of people age 55 and over," he observed. "But the marketing engines are in the hands of people who are thirty-somethings who are interested in selling to others like themselves." "Shopping Shift: Interview with Pico Underhill," *PBS News Hour,* April 24, 2009.

4. William Hupp, "The Misunderstood Generation," *Advertising Age,* February 5, 2008.

5. Metlife Mature Market Institute, *Boomer Bookends: Insights into the Oldest and Youngest Boomers* (Westport, CT: Metlife Mature Market Institute, February 2008), 17.

6. "Widely Held Attitudes to Different Generations," Harris Interactive Survey, August 20, 2008, www.marketresearchworld.net/index.php?option= com_content&task=view&id=2243&Itemid=77.

7. Steve Slon, interview with the author, Washington, DC, February 15, 2007.

8. Joe Queenan, "Please Don't Call Us That!" AARP.org, www.aarp.org/ personal-growth/transitions/info-07–2010/what_not_to_call_boomers.html.

9. Charles Duhigg, "Six Decades at the Center of Attention, and Counting," *New York Times,* January 6, 2008.

10. Randall Stross, "Do Boomers Want a Web Home of Their Own?" *New York Times,* February 10, 2008.

11. See Paul Briand, "The Continued Rise—and Fall—of Boomer Sites," *Examiner.com,* July 13, 2009, www.examiner.com/baby-boomer-in-national/ the-continued-rise-and-fall-of-boomer-sites; also Tanika White, "Boomers Go Online to Stay Connected," *Baltimore Sun,* April 27, 2008.

12. Diana Wagman, "The Cancer Drug," *Los Angeles Times,* December 22, 2007.

13. Marc Fisher, interview with the author, Claremont, CA, February 28, 2007.

14. Bill Novelli, interview with the author, Washington, DC, December 5, 2007.

15. Karl Mannheim, "The Problem of Generations" [1923], in *Essays on the Sociology of Knowledge* (New York: Oxford University Press, 1952).

16. For an excellent and more detailed discussion of these related concepts, see Duane F. Alwin, Ryan J. McCammon, and Scott M. Hofer, "Studying Baby Boom Cohorts within a Demographic and Developmental Context: Conceptual and Methodological Issues," in *Baby Boomers Grow Up,* ed. Susan Krauss Whitbourne and Sherry L. Willis (Mahwah, NJ: Lawrence Erlbaum, 2006), 45–74. See also Harry R. Moody, "Controversy 11. Aging Boomers: Boom or Bust?" in *Aging: Concepts and Controversies,* 6th ed., ed. Harry R. Moody (Thousand Oaks, CA: Pine Forge Press/Sage Publications, 2010), 429–32.

17. Robert Binstock, "Older Voters and the 2008 Election," *Gerontologist* 49, no. 5 (2010): 697–701.

18. Mannheim, "Problem of Generations," 301.

19. See Pew Research Center, "The Millennials: Confident. Connected. Open to Change," February 24, 2010, http://pewsocialtrends.org/assets/pdf/ millennials-confident-connected-open-to-change.pdf. Metlife Mature Market Institute, Demographic Generational Profiles, 2010, http://www.metlife .com/mmi/research/generational-profiles.html#introduction.

20. Key studies include Landon Y. Jones, *Great Expectations: America and the Baby Boom Generation* (New York: Ballantine Books, 1980); Paul Light, *Baby Boomers* (New York: Norton, 1988); William Strauss and Neil Howe, *Generations: The History of America's Future, 1584 to 2069* (New York: William Morrow, 1991); Ken Dychtwald, *Age Power: How the 21st Century Will Be Ruled by the New Old* (New York: Jeremy Tarcher/Putnam 1999); Michael Gross, *My Generation: Fifty Years of Sex, Drugs, Rock, Revolution, Glamour, Greed, Valor, Faith, and Silicon Chips* (New York: HarperCollins, 2000); Diane Macunovich, *Birth Quake: The Baby Boom and Its Aftershocks* (Chicago: University of Chicago Press, 2002); Steve Gillon, *Boomer Nation: The Largest and Richest Generation Ever and How It Changed America* (New York: Free Press, 2004); Marc Fisher, *Something in the Air: Radio, Rock, and the Revolution That Shaped a Generation* (New York: Random House, 2006); J. Walker Smith and Ann Clurman, *Generation Ageless: How Baby Boomers Are Changing the Way We Live Today* (New York: HarperCollins, 2007); and a recent overview by Alan Greenblatt, "Aging Baby Boomers," *CQ Researcher* 17, no. 37 (October 19, 2007): 865–88.

21. Jones, *Great Expectations,* 33.

22. Strauss and Howe, *Generations,* 368.

23. Pew Research Center, "Millennials."

24. Light, *Baby Boomers;* Smith and Clurman, *Generation Ageless,* 20.

25. Strauss and Howe, *Generations,* 309.

26. Peter Travers, "Steven Spielberg," *Rolling Stone: 40th Anniversary Issue,* May 3–17, 2007, 94.

27. Gross, *My Generation,* 10.

28. Leonard Steinhorn, *The Greater Generation* (New York: St. Martin's Press/Thomas Crowne Books, 2006).

29. Gillon, *Boomer Nation,* 285.

30. Strauss and Howe, *Generations,* 421.

31. Jones, *Great Expectations,* 306.

32. Tom Wolfe, "The 'Me' Decade and the Third Great Awakening," *New York Magazine,* August 23, 1976, 26–40.

33. Light, *Baby Boomers,* 148.

34. Ibid., 197–98.

35. Ibid., 204.

36. Robert Putnam, *Bowling Alone* (New York: Simon and Schuster, 2000).

37. Carol Keegan et al., *Boomers at Midlife: The AARP Life Stage Study* (Washington, DC: AARP Knowledge Management, 2002). A 2004 follow-up survey reinforced these findings: "By and large boomers believe that they can shape their future and that what happens in the future mostly depends on them." Carol Keegan et al., *Boomers at Midlife, 2004: The AARP Life Stage Study* (Washington, DC: AARP Knowledge Management, 2004). There were some variations in these patterns by race, class, and education—but surprisingly few by gender. The attitudes of Older Boomers (aged forty-six to fifty-six) resembled those of Younger Boomers (age thirty-eight to forty-five) rather than those of respondents who were older than fifty-seven.

38. Smith and Clurman, *Generation Ageless,* 29.

39. Ibid., 124.

40. *The Metlife Report on Early Boomers* (Westport, CT: Metlife Mature Market Institute/Peter Francese LLC, September 2010).

41. Ibid.

42. Annamaria Lusardi and Olivia S. Mitchell, "Baby Boomer Retirement Security: The Roles of Planning, Financial Literacy, and Housing Wealth," Ann Arbor, Michigan, University of Michigan Retirement Research Center, 2006, www.pensionresearchcouncil.org/publications/pdf/boomer.pdf.

43. Metlife Mature Market Institute, "Highlights of the MetLife Study of Boomers: Ready to Launch," 2007, www.metlife.com/assets/cao/mmi/publications/consumer/mmi-consumer-publications-boomers-ready-launch-hlghts.pdf.

44. David Rosnick and Dean Baker, *The Wealth of the Baby Boom Cohorts after the Collapse of the Housing Bubble* (Washington, DC: Center for Economic and Policy Research, 2009); Moody's estimate cited in Susan Tompor, "Boomers See Retirement Slip Farther Away," *Detroit Free Press,* September 20, 2010.

45. Macunovich, *Birth Quake,* 31.

46. See Elizabeth Warren and Amelia Tiagi, *The Two-Income Trap* (New York: Basic Books, 2003).

47. Mary Elizabeth Hughes and Angela M. O'Rand, *The Lives and Times of Baby Boomers* (New York: Russell Sage Foundation and Population Reference Bureau, 2004).

48. William Frey, "IV: Age," in *The State of Metropolitan America: On the Front Lines of Demographic Transformation* (Washington, DC: Brookings Institution, 2010), 78; also Jack VanDerhei, "The Impact of the Recent Financial Crisis on 401(k) Account Balances," *Employee Benefit Research Institute Issue Brief*, no. 326 (February 2009).

49. *Baby Boomers Envision Retirement II* (Washington, DC: AARP, May 2004); Merrill Lynch, *The New Retirement Survey* (New York: Merrill Lynch, 2005).

50. The "Wealth Builders" (31 percent) had the highest average incomes ($84,000) and the highest average assets ($214,000) and were tied with "Leisure Lifers" for highest percent white (82 percent). Driven by desire for material success and security, they were the most likely to describe themselves as workaholics and least likely to try and reinvent themselves (16 percent), enhance their spiritual life (25 percent), or volunteer (23 percent) during retirement. The 18 percent of the sample who were "Empowered Trailblazers" were second in average income ($83,000) and average assets ($188,000—does not include home equity) and were 72 percent white. They looked forward to a very active retirement of travel, exercise, additional education, and "new directions" and were the most likely to contribute to social causes and charities. The 20 percent of respondents classified as "Anxious Idealists" had the third-highest average income ($66,000) and fourth-highest average assets ($176,000) and were 68 percent white. Though they were the most likely to believe in "putting others first" (53 percent) and wanted to leave a significant inheritance to family and charitable organizations, they were worried that they had not adequately provided for their retirement needs. Thirteen percent of sample respondents were classified as "Leisure Lifers," half of whom had already retired. They had the fourth-highest average income ($64,000) and the third-highest average assets ($176,000) and were tied with the "Wealth Builders" for the highest percentage of whites (82 percent). More than three-quarters defined retirement in terms of rest and relaxation; they were the least likely to continue working, even to make up for financial shortfalls. Instead, 94 percent of them felt that their generation was entitled to full Social Security benefits and looked to government entitlements and their savings to make ends meet in retirement. At the bottom were the "Stretched and Stressed," 18 percent of survey recipients; this group was 66 percent white and had an average income of $60,000 and assets averaging $60,000.

51. Two more studies also segment boomers in terms of retirement dreams and general outlook. In *Generation Ageless*, Smith and Clurman's 2006 telephone survey sample of 1,023 boomers delineated six segments in terms of "future dreams." The "Re-activists" (15 percent) desired to remain active or reengage with social movements; they were the wealthiest, with 36 percent having an annual household income above $100,000. The "Disconnected" (8 percent) were sympathetic to the aims of the "Re-activists" but were more passive, preferring to tend to their own comfort; 35 percent had household incomes above $100,000. The "Sideliners" (20 percent) were more aloof and self-involved; 30 percent had incomes above $100,000. The "Maximizers" (15 percent) wanted to live life to the fullest, staying active and involved and accumulating experiences; 24 percent earned above $100,000. The "Straight Arrows" (33 percent) lived by traditional values and religion; 24 percent of them earned $100,000 or more. Finally, the "Due Diligents" (10 percent) were more cautious and wanted to enjoy "safe adventures," in part, perhaps, because only 18 percent earned $100,000 or more.

A 2006 Focalyst/AARP nationally representative sample survey of thirty-five thousand respondents over age forty-five yielded five segments structured more strongly by age and gender. "Dynamic Go-Getters" were the youngest (in their forties), wealthiest (average household income of $106,141), and best educated (71 percent college graduates). "Comfortable Everyman" was the second wealthiest (average household income of $99,737) and second best educated (45 percent college graduates) category, composed of almost exclusively age fifty-something men. Their counterpart was an almost all-female third boomer segment, "Today's Earth Mothers," socially and environmentally conscious women in their fifties; 37 percent had a college degree, and their average household income was $70,157. The "Stretched 40-Somethings" were just that: "average" working- and middle-class men and women (average household income $51,034) who were struggling to make ends meet; only 4 percent had college degrees. At the bottom were the "Downtrodden," individuals and couples in their fifties; 37 percent of them were college graduates, and they had an average household income of $37,050. "The Focalyst View Syndicated Report," Fall 2006, obtainable from www .focalyst.com.

52. Emilio Pardo, interview with the author, Washington, DC, June 15, 2006.

53. Richard Katz, telephone interview with the author, January 20, 2007.

54. Carleen MacKay, telephone interview with the author, November 21, 2006. See also Carleen MacKay, Phil Neubold, and Brad Taft, *Return of the Boomers: A Leader's Guide* (Scottsdale, AZ: Cambridge Media, LLC, 2008).

55. Andrew Johnson, telephone interview with the author, January 26, 2007.

2. OLD AGE IN A NEW SOCIETY

Chapter epigraphs are from C. Wright Mills, *White Collar* (New York: Oxford University Press, 1950); Robert Reich, *Supercapitalism* (New York: Alfred A. Knopf, 2007). The section epigraph is an anonymous Web post quoted in Jane Gross's "Single, Childless and 'Downright Terrified,'" *New York Times,* July 29, 2008.

1. C. Wright Mills, *White Collar* (New York: Oxford University Press, 1950).

2. Robert Reich, *Supercapitalism* (New York: Alfred A. Knopf, 2007).

3. See Alan Berube et al., *State of Metropolitan America: On the Front Lines of Demographic Transformation* (Washington, DC: Brookings Institution, 2010).

4. Fareed Zakaria, *The Post-American World* (New York: Norton, 2008).

5. Peggy Noonan, "Brave New World," *Wall Street Journal,* June 13, 2008.

6. David Shribman, "Today's Median Age Voters Grew Up in a Different America," *Real Clear Politics,* January 19, 2008.

7. Mathew Continetti, "Out with the Old: Don't Trust a Congressman over the Age of 50," *Weekly Standard,* May 31, 2010.

8. Roberta Garner, *Social Movements and Ideologies* (New York: McGraw Hill, 1996), 86–92.

9. Ibid., 93–99. See also Ben Wattenberg, *Fewer* (Chicago: Ivin R. Dee, 2004); Phillip Longman, *The Empty Cradle* (New York: New America Books/ Basic Books, 2004).

10. Mark Penn, "The Declining Soccer Mom," *Wall Street Journal,* October 7, 2009.

11. Jacob Hacker, *The Great Risk Shift* (New York: Oxford University Press, 2006).

12. Ibid., 6.

13. Reich, *Supercapitalism,* 126.

14. "Big Picture Series: Minnesota Voters Weigh Candidates' Economic Plans," *PBS News Hour,* January 29, 2008.

15. "Retirement and Medical Bills Top Financial Worries," *Employee Benefit News,* April 29, 2010, http://ebn.benefitnews.com/news/ retirement-medical-bills-top-financial-worries.

16. Matt Greenwald, interview with the author, Washington, DC, September 13, 2007.

17. Geoffrey Sanzenbacher, *Estimating Pension Coverage Using Different Data Sets,* Issue in Brief, no. 51 (Boston: Boston College Center for Retirement Research, August 2006).

18. See Stephan Fitch, "Gilt-Edged Pensions," *Forbes,* February 16, 2009. See also "Majority of Fortune 100 Companies Offer Only Defined Contribution Plans to New Salaried Employees," press release, Watson Wyatt Worldwide, May 11, 2009, www.watsonwyatt.com/render.asp?catid=1&id=21177; Sandra Block, "Traditional Company Pensions Are Going Away Fast," *USA Today,* May 21, 2009.

19. Employee Benefit Research Institute, "Retirement Trends in the United States over the Past Quarter Century," Factsheet, June 2007, www.ebri.org/pdf/publications/facts/0607fact.pdf.

20. Metlife Mature Market Institute, "Boomers Ready to Launch: Metlife Mature Market Institute Takes First Look at the Baby Boomers Turning 62," December 27, 2007, www.metlife.com/assets/cao/mmi/publications/mmi-pressroom/mmi-press-releases-boomers-ready-to-launch1226.pdf.

21. Fidelity Research Institute, *Fidelity Research Institute Retirement Index,* Research Insights Brief (Boston: Fidelity Research Institute, March 2007).

22. Jack VanDerhei, Sarah Holden, Craig Copeland, and Luis Alonso, "401K Plan Asset Allocation, Account Balances and Loan Activity in 2006," *Employee Benefit Research Institute Issue Brief,* no. 308 (August 2007).

23. Ruth Helman, Mathew Greenwald and Associates, Jack VenDerhei, and Craig Copeland, "The Retirement System in Transition: The 2007 Retirement Confidence Survey," *Employee Benefit Research Institute Issue Brief,* no. 304 (April 2007).

24. Thomas Kostigen, "The Inheritance Bust," Marketwatch, February 5, 2008, www.marketwatch.com/story/big-baby-boomer-inheritances-going-bust.

25. Fidelity Investments, "Fidelity Investments Couples Retirement Study: Executive Summary," June 2009, http://multivu.prnewswire.com/mnr/fidelity/38691/docs/38691-NEWExecSum_Couples2009_060509FINAL.pdf.

26. Scholars at the UCLA Center for Policy Research have authored a number of papers on Latino baby boomers, including Zachery D. Gassoumis, Kathleen H. Wilber, and Fernando Torres-Gil, *Latino Baby Boomers: A Hidden Population,* Policy Brief No. 3 (Los Angeles: UCLA Center for Policy Research on Aging, July 2008).

27. *Baby Boomers Envision Their Retirement* (Washington, DC: AARP, February 1999); *Baby Boomers Envision Retirement II* (Washington, DC: AARP, May 2004); Merrill Lynch, *The New Retirement Survey* (New York: Merrill Lynch, 2005).

28. Alicia H. Munnell, Mauricio Soto, Anthony Webb, Francesca Golub-Sass, and Dan Muldoon, *A New National Retirement Risk Index,* Issue in Brief, no. 48 (Boston: Boston College Center for Retirement Research, June 2006).

29. Alicia Munnell, Mauricio Soto, Anthony Webb, Francesca Golub-Sass, and Dan Muldoon, *Health Care Costs Drive Up the National Retirement Risk Index,* Issue in Brief, no. 8–3 (Boston: Boston College Center for Retirement Research, February 2008.

30. Carla Fried, "Have You Budgeted $250,000 for Health Care in Retirement?" CBS Moneywatch, March 23, 2010, http://moneywatch.bnet.com/retirement-planning/blog/retirement-beat/have-you-budgeted-250000-for-health-care-in-retirement/469/. See also Richard W. Johnson and Corin Mommaerts, *Will Health Care Costs Bankrupt Aging Boomers?* (Washington, DC: Urban Institute, February 2010). They predict that median, annual real out-of-pocket costs for Americans over age sixty-five will double (in 2008 dollars) from $2,600 in 2010 to $6,200 in 2040.

31. G. Smolka, L. Purvis, and C. Figueiredo, *Health Coverage among 50–64 Year Olds,* Data Digest (Washington, DC: AARP Policy Institute, 2007).

32. Fidelity Research Institute, *Fidelity Research Institute Retirement Index;* Kenneth Greene, "Spending and Spending Some More: Expenses in Later Life Are Proving to Be Bigger and More Unpredictable Than Many Retirees Anticipated," *Wall Street Journal,* May 12, 2007.

33. Heather Stern, telephone interview with the author, December 20, 2007.

34. Victoria Stagg Elliot, "Older Baby Boomers Sicker, Using More Care Than Earlier Generations," American Medical Association, Amednews.com, April 19, 2010, www.ama-assn.org/amednews/2010/04/19/bisb0419.htm. See also Virginia Fried and Amy B. Bernstein, *Health Care Utilization among Adults Aged 55–64 Years: How Has It Changed over the Past 10 Years?* Data Brief No. 32 (Hyattsville, MD: National Center for Health Statistics, 2010); Rob Stein, "Baby Boomers Appear to Be Less Healthy Than Parents," *Washington Post,* April 20, 2007.

35. Ibid.

36. U.S. Census Bureau, *Fertility of American Women: 2006,* Current Population Reports, P20–558 (Washington, DC, August 2008).

37. William Frey, *Mapping the Growth of Older America: Seniors and Boomers in the Early 21st Century,* Living Cities Census Series (Washington, DC: Brookings Institution, May 2007).

38. Jonathan Peterson, "A New Industry of Caregivers," *Los Angeles Times,* January 6, 2008.

39. Elizabeth Marquardt, "The New Alone," *Washington Post,* January 28, 2008, B1.

40. John Gist and Carlos Figueiredo, *In Their Dreams: What Will Boomers Inherit?* Data Digest (Washington, DC: AARP Public Policy Institute, May 2006); see also Eduardo Porter, "Inherit the Wind; There's Little Else Left," *New York Times,* March 26, 2006; Kelly K. Spors, "Counting on Getting an Inheritance? Better Make Other Plans," *Wall Street Journal,* October, 26, 2005; and Mitja Ng-Baumhacki, John Gist, and Carlos Figueiredo, *Pennies from Heaven,* Data Digest (Washington, DC: AARP Public Policy Institute, 2003).

41. Kostigen, "Inheritance Bust."

42. See William Frey and C.D. Ross, *America's Demography in the New Century: Aging Baby Boomers and New Immigrants as Major Players,* Policy Brief (Santa Monica, CA: Milken Institute, 2000); William H. Frey, *America's Regional Demographics in the '00s Decade: The Role of Seniors, Boomers and New Minorities,* Special Report (New York: Research for Housing America, 2006).

43. Sam Roberts, "New Demographic Racial Gap Emerges," *New York Times,* May 17, 2007.

44. Sam Roberts, "Minorities Often a Majority of the Population under 20," *New York Times,* August 7, 2008; see also William Frey, "Race and Ethnicity," in Berube et al., *State of Metropolitan Metro America.*

45. Dennis Cauchon, "Generation Gap? About $200,000," *USA Today,* May 20, 2007.

46. Julia B. Isaacs, Isabel V. Sawhill, and Ron Haskins, *Getting Ahead or Losing Ground: Economic Mobility in America* (Washington, DC: Economic Mobility Project/Brookings Institution, 2008).

47. Robert D. Putnam, "*E Pluribus Unum:* Diversity and Community in the Twenty-first Century: The 2006 Johan Skytte Prize Lecture," *Scandinavian Political Studies* 30, no. 2 (2007): 151.

48. See Kevin Starr, *Golden Dreams: California in an Age of Abundance, 1950–1963* (New York: Oxford University Press, 2009).

49. Cathleen Decker, "Pat Brown's California Takes a Beating in Sacramento," *Los Angeles Times,* July 26, 2009.

50. Shana Alex Lavarreda, E. Richard Brown, Livier Cabezas, and Dylan H. Roby, *Number of Uninsured Jumped to More Than Eight Million from 2007 to 2009*, UCLA Health Policy Research Brief (Los Angeles: UCLA Center for Health Policy Research, March 2010).

51. Steve Lopez, "At a Free Clinic, Scenes from the Third World," *Los Angeles Times,* August 16, 2009.

52. Cathleen Decker, "Down but Not Out, Imperial County Looks to a Better Future," *Los Angeles Times,* May 9, 2010.

53. Mark Baldassare, Dean Bonner, Sonja Petek, and Nicole Wilcoxon, *Californians and Their Government* (San Francisco: Public Policy Institute of California, January 2010). Response of "voters" is from Evan Halper, "State Voters Largely Back Health Law," *Los Angeles Times,* April 4, 2010.

54. Robert J. Samuelson, "California's Reckoning—and Ours," *Newsweek,* August 3, 2009.

55. Peter Schrag, *Paradise Lost* (Berkeley: University of California Press, 1998); and *California: America's High-Stakes Experiment* (Berkeley: University of California Press, 2006); Dowell Myers, *Immigrants and Boomers: Forging a New Social Contract for the Future of America* (New York: Russell Sage Foundation, 2007). See also Mark Baldassare, *California's Exclusive Electorate* (San Francisco: Public Policy Institute of California, 2004).

56. Dan Walters, "California Faces Huge Upheaval," *Sacramento Bee,* May 4, 2008.

57. See Justin Berton, "Whites in State 'Below the Replacement' Level," *San Francisco Chronicle,* June 5, 2010.

58. Dowell Myers and John Pitkin, "The New Place of Birth Profile of Los Angeles and California Residents in 2010," University of Southern California School of Policy, Planning and Development, Los Angeles, March 2010, www.usc.edu/schools/sppd/research/popdynamics/pdf/Myers_Pitkin_Placeof-BirthReport_033110.pdf. The figure on the city of Los Angeles is from George Will, "Trickle Down Misery," *Newsweek,* May 17, 2010.

59. Jeffrey L. Rabin, "Shifting Demographics: Immigrants Could Be Key to Boomers' Security," interview with Dowell Myers, February 27, 2007.

60. California Department of Education Data and Statistics, "Public School Summary Statistics, 2005–06," June 2006, www.cde.ca.gov/ds/sd/cb/sums05.asp; Terence Chea, "Budget Crisis Forces Deep Cuts at California Schools," Associated Press, June 21, 2009, http://apnews.myway.com/article/20090621/D98V7T001.htm.

61. Jay P. Greene and Marcus A. Winters, "Public High School Graduation and College Readiness Rates: 1991–2002," Education Working Paper No. 8, Center for Civic Innovation, Manhattan Institute, New York, February 2005.

62. Cari Tuna, "University of California Plans to Slash Spending," *Wall Street Journal,* May 18, 2010.

63. Jack Citrin, a University of California, Berkeley professor with expertise on California state politics, maintains that Prop. 13's effects were not as drastic as Schrag suggests. "In the past 30 years, California, once a high tax and high services state in the rankings of American states, moved down both ladders and now is in the middle of both tax and overall spending rankings." Jack Citrin, "Proposition 13 and the Transformation of California Government," *California Journal of Politics and Policy* 1, no. 1 (2009), www.bepress.com/cjpp/vol1/iss1/16.

64. Schrag, *California,* 18.

65. Steve Lopez, "Assembly Leader Sees Opportunity in the State's Crisis," *Los Angeles Times,* December 24, 2008. Kerkorian's views were substantiated a month later in another grim report by the California Faculty Association, Thomas G. Mortenson's "California at the Edge of a Cliff: The Failure to Invest in Public Higher Education is Crushing the Economy and Crippling Our Kids' Future," Report to the California Faculty Association, January 2009, www.postsecondary.org/archives/Reports/CAattheEdge1.pdf.

66. Mark Baldassare, *California's Post-partisan Future* (San Francisco: Public Policy Institute of California, 2008).

67. Joel Kotkin, "Sundown for California," *American Magazine,* November 12, 2008, www.american.com/archive/2008/november-december-magazine/sundown-forcalifornia. See also Kotkin's "Death of the Dream," *Newsweek,* March 2, 2009, "Can California Make a Comeback?" *Forbes,* May 26, 2009, and "California after the Deluge," lecture at Claremont McKenna College, Athenaeum series, January 29, 2008. For a similar view by a longtime California observer, see Harold Meyerson, "California: A Dream Diminished," *Washington Post,* July 1, 2009. (See also "Traffic, Schools, Job Loss Cited as Reasons for Wanting to Leave L.A.," *Los Angeles Times,* July 10, 2009—as well as numerous "comments" emphasizing a topic not explicitly addressed in the article: illegal immigration.)

68. Joel Kotkin, "Boomer Economy Stunting Growth in Northern California," *Forbes,* November 16, 2009, www.forbes.com/2009/11/16/california-boomers-economy-opinion.htm.

69. Pat Morrison, "Making History" (interview with Kevin Starr), *Los Angeles Times,* July 11, 2009.

70. Conor Dougherty, "U.S. Nears Racial Milestone," *Wall Street Journal,* June 11, 2010.

71. William Frey, "Three Americas: How Migration Is Changing America," lecture at Claremont McKenna College, Athenaeum series, April 20, 2004; Also Frey, *America's Regional Demographics* and *Mapping the Growth.*

72. Frey, "Race and Ethnicity."

73. See Eric Bailey, "Cries for Reform of California Government Come from All Sides," *Los Angeles Times,* July 14, 2009; Kevin O'Leary, "How California's Fiscal Woes Began: A Crisis 30 Years in the Making," *Time,* July 1, 2009; Joel Fox, "Proposition 13 Isn't the Problem," *Los Angeles Times,* July 9, 2009; John Vasconcellos, "How Did California Get into This Mess?" *Los Angeles Times,* July 10, 2009.

74. In early 2010, the movement for a constitutional convention suffered a temporary setback when Repair California could obtain only a fraction of the signatures needed to schedule a November ballot initiative. See "A Political Triple Whammy," editorial, *Los Angeles Times,* February 16, 2010.

75. Myers, *Immigrants and Boomers.*

76. Schrag, *California,* 244.

77. The success of these populist "rebellions" relies on the fact that California's frequent voters and "special election voters" tend to be disproportionately white, college-educated, middle-class homeowners over age fifty. See Mark Baldassare, Dean Bonner, Jennifer Paluch, and Sonja Petek, *Californians and Their Government* (San Francisco: Public Policy Institute of California, May 2009).

78. Boomers and those over sixty-five are most opposed to illegal immigration—in contrast to younger Americans. See Damien Cave, "A Generation Gap over Immigration," *New York Times,* May 17, 2010. This article is heavily based on the chapters by William Frey in Berube et al., *State of Metropolitan America.*

79. Ronald Brownstein, "The Gray and the Brown: The Generational Mismatch," *National Journal,* July 24, 2010.

80. See Pew Research Center, "Limbaugh Holds onto His Niche—Conservative Men," February 3, 2009, http://pewresearch.org/pubs/1102/limbaugh-audience-conservative-men.

81. On the quickening drumbeat for Proposition 13 reform, see Bill Stahl, "Assessing Proposition 13," *Los Angeles Times,* May 29, 2008; Michael Rothfield

and Eric Bailey, "California's Budget Fiasco Legacy Could Be Reform," *Los Angeles Times,* February 20, 2009; Jerry Robert and Phil Trounsline, "Why California Can't Be Governed," *Los Angeles Times,* June 25, 2009; O'Leary, "How California's Fiscal Woes Began," Fox, "Proposition 13 Isn't the Problem"; Vasconcellos, "How Did California Get into This Mess?"; Jon Chang, "Group Airs Proposals for California Government Overhaul," *Sacramento Bee,* August 15, 2009.

82. Again, see Berton, "Whites in State." From 2005 to 2007, California again became a net "exporter" of residents to other states. According to California demographer Joel Kotkin ("Death of the Dream"), the net outflow should reach 200,000 by 2010. Kotkin further admits that rising numbers might even be higher if the real estate recession hadn't dashed the dreams of many near-retirees hoping to "cash out" at peak prices and then move to locales with lower costs of living. See also Mike Swift, "Boomers Leaving Golden State," *San Jose Mercury News,* May 1, 2008; "California, Here We Come," *Washington Examiner,* July 1, 2009; Michael R. Blood, "Go East, Young Man? Californians Look for the Exit," Associated Press, January 13, 2009; Kotkin, "Sundown for California."

83. Teresa Watanabe, "Naturalized Citizens Are Poised to Reshape California's Political Landscape," *Los Angeles Times,* May 11, 2009.

84. Allan Hoffenblum, "California's Plummeting GOP Registration," April 14, 2009, www.foxandhoundsdaily.com/blog/allan-hoffenblum/californias-plummeting-gop-registration.

3. BOOMERS' SENIOR POWER POTENTIAL

1. Interview with the author, Washington, DC, February 13, 2007.

2. "New AARP Survey Shows Public Strongly Opposes Social Security Private Accounts," October 24, 2006, http://www-alpha.aarp.org/aarp/articles/pulse_poll_social_security.html.

3. Greenberg, Quinlin, Rosner Research, *2005 Likely Voter Survey* (Washington, DC: Greenberg, Quinlin, Rosner Research Inc., 2005).

4. David Court, Diana Farrell, and John E. Forsyth, "Serving Aging Baby Boomers," *McKinsey Quarterly,* no. 4 (2007): 105.

5. Andrew Johnson, telephone interview with the author, January 26, 2007.

6. William Frey, "Race, Immigration and America's Changing Electorate," in *Red, Blue and Purple America: The Future of Election Demographics,* ed. Ruy Teixeira (Washington, DC: Brookings Institution Press, 2008), 85.

7. In an analysis of voting data, Duane Alwin found that in the 1970s more than 70 percent felt the government would do what was right; by 1994 only 20 percent thought so. Though boomers were once somewhat more favorable toward government efforts to help minorities, they joined an overall trend in declining support for such programs: 45 percent of boomers supported affirmative action in the 1970s; by 1994, fewer than 25 percent did so. Politically independent boomers moved toward Republican Party identification—from 12 percent in the 1970s to 30 percent in 1994. Alwin concluded that although boomers might have remained liberal on a range of social issues, they might also accelerate broader trends toward conservatism. See Duane Alwin, "The Political Impact of the Baby Boom: Are There Persistent Generational Differences in Political Beliefs and Behavior?" *Generations* 22, no. 1 (1998): 46–54.

8. "John B. Williamson, "Political Activism and the Aging of the Baby Boom," *Generations* 22, no. 1 (1998: 55–59). Susan A. MacManus in *Young v. Old: Generational Combat in the 21st Century* (Boulder, CO: Westview Press, 1996) also acknowledged the growth and importance of old-age organizations and their location near national centers of power in Washington, DC.

McManus examined generational cohesion and differences across a range of attitudinal and behavioral variables. The results were more suggestive than definitive. In terms of generational attitudes toward taxing and spending policies, MacManus found that "all age groups express a preference for politics that are (or would be) most advantageous to them at that point in their lives. No one age-group holds exclusive rights to being labeled 'greedy' or 'self-centered'" (244). She found that older voters do indeed register and vote more than the young. Older voters were more likely to contact public officials, but younger and middle-aged voters were more likely to be active in signing and circulating petitions. Older Americans were far more likely to contribute to PACs than the young. Older Americans tended to self-identify as Democrats, while higher proportions of the young were Republicans—though there were trends in both groups toward identification as independents.

MacManus predicts that generational political differences will widen in the future, especially on health care policies, criminal justice, and moral and social issues. (On the latter topic, the young tend to favor individual rights over societal protection, while older Americans reverse preferences.) Policy proposals may take on an "us-against-them" quality, and "younger cohorts will attempt to guard against tax structures that would place heavy burdens on them and to fight for a fair share of scarce resources for themselves and their children. Equity concerns will likely supplant efficiency issues in the 1990s and beyond" (245).

9. Carol Keegan et al., *Boomers at Midlife: The AARP Life Stage Study* (Washington, DC: AARP Knowledge Management, 2002), and *Boomers at Midlife, 2004: The AARP Life Stage Study* (Washington, DC: AARP Knowledge Management, 2004).

10. Merrill Lynch, *The New Retirement Survey* (New York: Merrill Lynch, 2005). In a related matter, boomers and other Americans are showing increasing support for government-assisted efforts to support universal health care access. A 2006 AARP poll of voters over age forty-two found that health care was a top political concern and that 78 percent favored minimum health insurance benefits for all Americans. *AARP National Member Survey about 2006 Election Issues* (Washington, DC: AARP Knowledge Management, June 2006).

11. Andrea Louise Campbell, *How Policies Make Citizens* (Princeton: Princeton University Press, 2003).

12. Ibid., 2.

13. Robert Binstock, "Older People and Voting Participation," *Gerontologist* 40, no. 1 (2000): 18–39.

14. James H. Schulz and Robert H. Binstock, *Aging Nation: The Economics and Politics of Growing Older in America* (New York: Praeger, 2006).

15. Ibid., 207. Binstock has discerned the imprint of 1950s period effects upon one group of voters aged sixty-five to seventy-four, an "Eisenhower cohort." They formed their early political allegiances during the Eisenhower presidency of the 1950s; and that cohort has since tended to disproportionately favor Republican candidates in presidential elections, more so than voters slightly older or slightly younger. Other than that, however, the Eisenhower cohort and other senior voters have not responded as a distinctive voting bloc even in the few elections when age policy issues were salient. See Robert Binstock, "Older Voters and the 2008 Election," *Gerontologist* 49, no. 5 (2010): 697–701.

16. See Ralph H. Turner and Lewis M. Killian, *Collective Behavior,* 3rd ed. (Englewood Cliffs, NJ: Prentice-Hall, 1987); also Gary T. Marx and Douglas McAdam, *Collective Behavior and Social Movements: Process and Structure* (Englewood Cliffs, NJ: Prentice-Hall, 1994).

17. Alan Wolfe, *One Nation after All: What Americans Really Think about God, Country, Family, Racism, Welfare, Immigration, Homosexuality, Work, the Right, the Left, and Each Other* (New York: Viking Press, 1998).

18. Peter Beinart, "The New Liberal Order," *Time,* November 13, 2008.

19. Steve Vogel, "Age Discrimination Claims Jump, Worrying EEOC, Worker Advocates," *Washington Post,* July 16, 2009. See also Jennifer Levitz and Philip Shishkin, "More Workers Cite Age Bias after Layoffs," *Wall Street Journal,* March 10, 2009.

20. David G. Savage, "Supreme Court Makes Age-Bias Suits Harder to Win," *Los Angeles Times,* June 19, 2009.

21. "Age Discrimination," *New York Times,* July 7, 2009.

22. See a detailed analysis of the poll in Ronald Brownstein's "Back to Basics," *National Journal,* September 11, 2010. Original poll data at www .nationaljournal.com/njonline/ASNJHeartlandMonitorVITolplines.pdf.

23. Annie Gowen, "Lying Low after a Layoff," *Washington Post,* August 12, 2009.

24. Anne Hull, "Squeaking By on $300,000," *Washington Post,* August 16, 2009.

25. John J. Heldrich Center for Workforce Development, "The Anguish of Unemployment," Rutgers University, September 2009, www.heldrich .rutgers.edu/sites/default/files/content/Heldrich_Work_Trends_Anguish_ Unemployment.pdf.

26. "Agency Files Age Discrimination Suit against AT&T," *AARP Bulletin Today,* August 20, 2009.

27. AARP, *A Changing Political Landscape as One Generation Replaces Another* (Washington, DC: AARP Knowledge Management, 2004), 14. The AARP report recognized that boomers' politics had been conditioned by their generational history—one that differed markedly from that of their GI-generation parents. Not surprisingly, boomers identified the Vietnam War and the movements for civil rights and women's rights as shaping their political worldview; older GIs saw World War II and the Great Depression as their formative experiences. Boomers' heritage of protest and skepticism is reflected in findings that (1) more boomers than GIs were political independents (39 vs. 24 percent); (2) more boomers than GIs saw the need for a strong third party (56 vs. 37 percent); and (3) boomers were more likely to select candidates by stance on key issues, whereas GIs tended to emphasize candidates' personal qualities.

28. Ibid., 13.

29. One of the most cited recent studies on the polarization of the occupational structure is David Autor, "The Polarization of Job Opportunities in the U.S. Labor Market," Center for American Progress and the Hamilton Project, April 2010, www.americanprogress.org/issues/2010/04/pdf/ job_polarization.pdf.

30. The liberal/Democratic tilt of liberal arts college and university faculties is well known. More recently, the Pew Research Center took the political pulse of a sample of research scientists: only 6 percent were Republican; 55 percent were Democrats, and 32 percent were Independents. See Pew Research Center, "Public Praises Science; Scientists Fault Public, Media," Washington, DC, July 9, 2009, http://people-press.org/reports/pdf/528.pdf.

31. Robert Putnam, "The Growing Class Gap," *Pittsburgh Post Gazette*, April 28, 2008.

32. Christopher Lasch, *The Revolt of the Elites* (New York: Norton, 1995), 35.

33. Robert Kaplan, *An Empire Wilderness: Travels into America's Future* (New York: Random House, 1998), 35.

34. Ibid., 73.

35. Ibid., 101.

36. David Halberstam, *The Best and the Brightest* (New York: Random House, 1972).

37. Joan Didion, *The Year of Magical Thinking* (New York: Alfred A. Knopf, 2003), 98.

38. As Beinart ("New Liberal Order") put it very well: "The biggest potential land mine in the Obama coalition isn't the culture war or foreign policy; it's nationalism. On a range of issues, from global warming to immigration to trade to torture, college-educated liberals want to integrate more deeply America's economy, society and values with the rest of the world's. They want to make it easier for people and goods to legally cross America's borders, and they want global rules that govern how much America can pollute the atmosphere and how it conducts the war on terrorism. They believe that ceding some sovereignty is essential to making America prosperous, decent and safe. When it comes to free trade, immigration and multilateralism, though, downscale Democrats are more skeptical. In the future, the old struggle between freedom and order may play itself out on a global scale, as liberal internationalists try to establish new rules for a more interconnected planet and working-class nationalists protest that foreign bureaucrats threaten America's freedom."

39. Peter Brown, "Like Affirmative Action, Arizona Law Splits Elites and the Public," *Wall Street Journal*, May 20, 2010.

40. Peggy Noonan, "Try a Little Tenderness," *Wall Street Journal*, February 2, 2008.

41. Stanley B. Greenberg and James Carville, "Solving the Paradox of 2004," Washington, DC, Democracy Corps, November 9, 2004.

42. See, for example, Thomas Frank, *What's the Matter with Kansas? How Conservatives Won the Heart of America* (New York: Henry Holt, 2004).

43. Alan Abramowitz and Ruy Teixeira, "The Decline of the White Working Class and the Rise of a Mass Upper Middle Class," in Teixeira, *Red, Blue and Purple America*.

44. Ibid. This finding is indicative of what Abramowitz and Teixeira describe as tensions within a "mass upper middle class" between managers, who still lean Republican, and highly educated professionals, who are trending Democratic.

45. See David Brady, Benjamin Sosnaud, and Steven M. Frenk, "The Shifting and Diverging White Working Class in the U.S. Presidential Elections, 1972–2004," *Social Science Research* 38, no. 1 (2009): 118–33.

46. See Lydia Saad, "White Gender Gap in Obama Approval Widens with Education," Gallup Polls, May 21, 2010, www.gallup.com/poll/128261/white-gender-gap-obama-approval-widens-education.aspx; Ronald Brownstein, "Two Suburbs, Two Views of Obama," *National Journal,* July 10, 2010; Joel Kotkin, "The Democrats' Middle Class Problem," *Politico,* July 14, 2010, www.politico.com/news/stories/0710/39675.html.

47. Andrew Sullivan, "Good-Bye to All That," *Atlantic Monthly,* December 2007, 40–54.

48. Caroline Kennedy, "A President Like My Father," op-ed, *New York Times,* January 27, 2008.

49. Susan Eisenhower, "Why I'm Backing Obama," op-ed, *Washington Post,* February 2, 2008.

50. Matt Bai, "Back-Room Choices," *New York Times Magazine,* February 3, 2008.

51. Morley Winograd and Michael D. Hais, "The Boomers Had Their Day, Make Way for the Millennials," *Washington Post,* February 3, 2008.

52. Roger Cohen, "Obama's Youth-Driven Movement," *New York Times,* January 28, 2008.

53. Bill Clinton, interview, *Charlie Rose Show,* December 14, 2007, www.charlierose.com/view/interview/8836#frame_top.

54. Jay Cost, "Review of Obama's Voting Coalition, Pts I-IV," May 27, 2008, www.realclearpolitics.com/horseraceblog/2008/05/a_review_of_obamas_voting_coalition_1.html.

55. Among white voters age eighteen to twenty-nine, the Clinton-Obama split was 53 to 47 percent; among voters thirty to forty-four, Clinton increased the gap 61 to 34 percent; among those forty-five to sixty (the boomer

demographic), Clinton's lead widened still further, 68 to 31 percent; and for those voters over age sixty, Clinton had a decisive margin over Obama of 75 to 23 percent. Ibid.

A Brookings Institution demographer offered a somewhat parallel analysis, noting that Clinton had the advantage in the "old white belt" of "slow growing battlegrounds" including much of the Great Lakes and Midwest, while Obama had the advantage in the more diverse fast-growing battlegrounds such as Florida and many of the mountain states, such as Colorado, Nevada, and New Mexico. See Tom Edsall, "Is Obama or Clinton the Better General Election Candidate?" www.realclearpolitics.com/articles/2008/03/is_obama_or_clinton_the-better.html, March 12, 2008.

56. CNN Exit Poll, November 5, 2008, www.cnn.com/ELECTION/2008/results/polls/#USP00P1.

57. Ibid.

58. Ronald Brownstein, "Obama and the Swells," *National Journal*, April 25, 2009.

59. Peter Wallstein, "Democrats Face Threat from Their Own Base," *Wall Street Journal*, May 19, 2010. See also Brownstein, "Two Suburbs," and Ronald Brownstein, "Obama's Electoral Headwinds," *National Journal*, September 11, 2010.

60. See Thomas Edsall, "The Obama Coalition," *Atlantic Monthly*, April, 2010.

61. Katherine Q. Seelye, "In Clinton vs. Obama, Age Is One of the Greatest Predictors," *New York Times*, April 22, 2008.

62. Chuck Todd and Sledon Gawiser, *How Obama Won* (New York: Vintage Books, 2009), 31.

63. Patrick Fisher, "The Age Gap in the 2008 Presidential Election," *Society* 47 (December 2009): 295–300.

64. Morley Winograd and Michael D. Hais, *Millennial Makeover: MySpace, YouTube, and the Future of American Politics* (New Brunswick: Rutgers University Press, 2008), 206.

65. Ibid., 210.

66. Thomas Friedman, "More (Steve) Jobs, Jobs, Jobs, Jobs," *New York Times*, January 23, 2010. See also James Oliphant and Kathleen Hennessey, "Obama's Electoral Coalition Is Crumbling," *Los Angeles Times*, September 11, 2010.

67. Cited in Peter Nicholas and Christi Parsons, "Obama's Midterm Task: Reenergize Voters," *Los Angeles Times*, July 13, 2010.

68. Matt Bai, "Midterms Are a Test for the Real Ground Game," *New York Times,* October 13, 2010.

69. Karen Tumulty, "Democrats Spend Big to Lure Obama's Minority and Young Voters Back to the Polls," *Washington Post,* June 20, 2010.

70. See Kate Zernike, *Boiling Mad: Inside Tea Party America* (New York: Times Books, 2010).

71. Kate Zernike and Megan Thee-Brenan, "Poll Finds Tea Party Backers Wealthier and More Educated," *New York Times,* April 14, 2010.

72. Pew Research Center, "The People and Their Government: Distrust, Discontent, Anger and Partisan Rancor," April 18, 2010, http://people-press. org/reports/pdf/606.pdf, 90–91.

73. "Polling the Tea Party," *New York Times,* April 14, 2010. Interactive feature: www.nytimes.com/interactive/2010/04/14/us/politics/20100414-tea-party-poll-graphic.html?ref=politics#tab=3.

74. Zernike and Thee-Brenan, "Poll Finds Tea Party." A subsequent Bloomberg national poll of Tea Party supporters found that 53 percent would consider raising the eligibility age for Medicare and 58 percent would consider similar action on Social Security—compared to 47 percent and 49 percent, respectively, of the general public. See www.bloomberg.com/news/2010–10–14/tea-party-s-economic-gloom-fuels-republican-election-momentum-poll-says.html.

4. CRASH LANDING FOR A SELF-CRITICAL GENERATION

The chapter epigraph is taken from Thomas J. Friedman, "Root Canal Politics," *New York Times,* May 8, 2010.

1. "Targeting Your 401(k)," *Wall Street Journal,* November 14, 2008.

2. Robert Samuelson, "A Darker Future for Us," *Newsweek,* November 10, 2008.

3. David M. Walker, "Call This a Crisis? Just Wait!" *Fortune*/CNN Money. com, October 30, 2008, and *Comeback America: Turning the Country Around and Restoring Fiscal Responsibility* (New York: Random House, 2009).

4. See Steven Erlanger, "Crisis Imperils Liberal Benefits Long Expected by Europeans," *New York Times,* May 22, 2010; also Mary Williams Walsh and Amy Schoenfeld, "Padded Pensions Add to New York Fiscal Woes," *New York Times,* May 20, 2010 (this includes assessments from a variety of pension experts in an accompanying section entitled "Room for Debate"); Mortimer Zuckerman, "The Bankrupting of America," *Wall Street Journal,* May 21, 2010;

Alan Blinder, "Return of the Bond Market Vigilantes," *Wall Street Journal*, May 20, 2010.

5. S. Kathi Brown, *A Year-End Look at the Economic Slowdown's Impact on Middle-Aged and Older Americans* (Washington, DC: AARP Knowledge Management, January 2009).

6. Greg Anrig and Millie Parekh, "The Impact of Housing and Investment Market Declines on the Wealth of Baby Boomers," Issue Brief, Century Foundation, August 2, 2010, http://tcf.org/publications/2010/7/the-impact-of-housing-and-investment-market-declines-on-the-wealth-of-baby-boomers/pdf.

7. Alicia H. Munnell and Dan Muldoon, *Are Retirement Savings Too Exposed to Market Risk?* Issue in Brief, no. 8–16 (Boston: Boston College Center for Retirement Research, October 2008).

8. Alicia H. Munnell, Anthony Webb, and Francesca Golub-Sass, *The National Retirement Risk Index: After the Crash,* Issue in Brief, no. 9–22 (Boston: Boston College Center for Retirement Research, October 2009), 7.

9. Obviously, the composition of the job tenure categories changed for people who remained with the same employer—or retired after more than thirty years on the job.

10. Jack VanDerhei, Sarah Holden, and Luis Alonso, "401(k) Plan Asset Allocation, Account Balances, and Loan Activity in 2008," *Employee Benefit Research Institute Issue Brief,* no. 335 (October 2009), 11–12.

11. "Change in Average Account Balances (by Age and Tenure) from January 1, 2008–December 31, 2009 among 401(k) Participants with Account Balances as of Dec. 31, 2007," Employee Benefits Research Institute, www.ebri.org/pdf/December%2031,%202009%20update%20full%20universe.pdf.

12. Jack VanDerhei and Craig Copeland, "The EBRI Retirement Readiness Rating; Retirement Income Preparation and Future Prospects," *Employee Benefit Research Institute Issue Brief,* no. 344 (July 2010). (The report uses the terms *Early Boomers* and *Late Boomers* and also defines Early Boomers as those born between 1948 and 1964, rather than the traditional birth range of 1946 to 1964.)

13. Alicia Munnell and Jean-Pierre Aubry, *Returns on 401(k) Assets by Cohort,* Issue in Brief, no. 10–6 (Boston: Boston College Center for Retirement Research, March 2010).

14. Peter Y. Hong, "Southern California Home Prices Rise Slightly in May," *Los Angeles Times,* June 18, 2009.

15. "Deutsche Bank Predicts 40% Drop in New York Home Prices," *Wall Street Journal,* June 16, 2009.

16. David Rosnick and Dean Baker, "The Wealth of the Baby Boom Cohorts after the Collapse of the Housing Bubble," Report, Center for Economic and Policy Research, Washington, DC, February 2009, www.cepr.net/documents/publications/baby-boomer-wealth-2009–02.pdf. (An Urban Institute study suggests that declining home values may be more of a psychological than an economic jolt; only about 6 percent of those aged fifty to sixty-five plan to use home equity to finance daily living expenses in retirement. Richard W. Johnson, Mauricio Soto, and Shela R. Zedlewski, "How Is the Economic Turmoil Affecting Older Americans?" Fact Sheet, Urban Institute, Washington, DC, October 2008, www.urban.org/UploadedPDF/411765_economic_turmoil.pdf.)

17. Tom Lauricella, "Retiring? Pay Off Your Mortgage," *Wall Street Journal,* August 6, 2009.

18. "Net Worth of Families Down Sharply," *New York Times,* March 12, 2009.

19. Federal Reserve Flow of Funds Accounts, March 11, 2010, www.federalreserve.gov/RELEASES/z1/20100311/.

20. "Net Worth of Families Down Sharply."

21. Jeffry M. Jones, "Boomers' Spending Like Other Generations', Down Sharply," Gallup Poll, August 27, 2009, www.gallup.com/poll/122546/boomers-spending-generations-down-sharply.aspx.

22. Barbara Butrica, Karen E. Smith, and Eric Toder, *How Will the Stock Market Collapse Affect Retirement Incomes?* Older Americans' Economic Security, no. 20 (Washington, DC: Urban Institute, June 2009).

23. Alan L. Gustman, Thomas L. Steinmeir, and Nahid Tabatabai, "What the Stock Market Decline Means for the Financial Security and Retirement Choices of the Near Retirement Population," Working Paper No. 15235, National Bureau of Economic Research, Washington, DC, October 2009, www.nber.org/papers/w15435.

24. See Richard Wolf, "Social Security Collectors Up 19%," *USA Today,* October 1, 2009.

25. Tony Pugh, "Social Security Surplus Hit by Joblessness, Early Retirement," *Miami Herald,* February 11, 2010, www.miamiherald.com/news/politics/AP/story/1475405.html.

26. Sandra Block, "Boomer Quandary," *USA Today,* March 11, 2008.

27. Kelly Evans and Sarah E. Needleman, "For Older Workers, a Reluctant Retirement," *Wall Street Journal,* December 8, 2009. See also AARP, "Last Decade Spelled Disaster for Older Workers," press release,

March 3, 2010, www.aarp.org/about-aarp/press-center/info-03–2010/last_decade_spelleddiasterforolderworkers.html.

28. Dennis Cauchon, "Employed See Tough Times, Too," *USA Today,* June 13, 2009.

29. U.S. Bureau of Labor Statistics, *Monthly Labor Report,* July 1, 2009; Sara E. Rix, "The Employment Situation, June, 2010: A Mixed Picture for Older Workers." Fact Sheet 195, AARP Public Policy Institute, July 2010, www.aarp.org/work/job-hunting/info-07–2010/fs195-economic.html. See also Emily Glazer, "Out of Work, Out of Options, and Over the Hill," *Wall Street Journal,* October 24, 2010. For a one-year follow-up of a small, nonscientific sample of unemployed boomers, see Michael Winerip, "Boomers in a Post-boom Economy," *New York Times,* March 1, 2009, and Michael Winerip, "Time, It Turns Out, Isn't on Their Side," *New York Times,* March 11, 2010.

30. "Poll: Less Job Security Is the 'New Normal,'" ABC News, June 15, 2009, http://abcnews.go.com/PollingUnit/Story?id=7802574&page=3.

31. Courtney Coile and Philip B. Levine, "The Market Crash and Mass Layoffs: How the Current Economic Crisis May Affect Retirement," Working Paper No. 15395, National Bureau of Economic Research, Washington, DC, October 2009, www.nber.org/papers/w15395.

32. Ruth Helman, Mathew Greenwald and Associates, Craig Copeland, and Jack VanDerhei, "The 2010 Retirement Confidence Survey: Confidence Stabilizing but Preparations Continue to Erode," *Employee Benefit Research Institute Issue Brief,* no. 340 (March 2010).

33. Towers Watson, "Older Worker Confidence in Retirement Security Drops Sharply, Watson Wyatt Survey Finds," press release, June 2, 2009, www.watsonwyatt.com/render.asp?catid=1&id=21316.

34. Steve French, "Boomer Opportunities: Trends among the Largest Demographic In America," paper presented at the National Conference on Aging/American Society on Aging Joint Annual Conference, Chicago, March 16, 2010.

35. Matt Ackerman, "Retirement Assets Surged 18% to $9.3 Trillion," *Employee Benefit News,* April 15, 2010.

36. Sarah N. Lynch, "Survey Says Household Stick with 401(k)s," *Wall Street Journal,* January 2, 2010.

37. Brennan and Stevens discussed these reports on PBS *Nightly Business Report,* January 8, 2010. See John Ameriks, Anna Madamba, and Stephen P. Utkus, *The Aftermath: Investor Attitudes in the Wake of the 2008–2009 Market Decline* (Valley Forge, PA: Vanguard Center for Retirement Research, October 2009);

Sarah Holden, John Sabelhaus, and Brian Reid, *Enduring Confidence in the 401(k) System: Investor Attitudes and Actions* (Washington, DC: Investment Company Institute, January 2010).

38. Theo Francis, "Retiree Annuities May Be Promoted by Obama Aides," *Businessweek,* January 8, 2010.

39. E. S. Browning, "Small Investors Flee Stocks, Changing Market Dynamics," *Wall Street Journal,* July 12, 2010. See also Graham Bowley, "In Striking Shift, Small Investors Flee Stock Market," *New York Times,* August 21, 2010.

40. Pew Research Center, "How the Great Recession Has Changed Life in America," report, Washington, DC, June 30, 2010, http://pewsocialtrends.org/pubs/759/how-the-great-recession-has-changed-life-in-america?utm_source=feedburner&utm_medium=feed&utm_campaign=Feed:+pewsocialtrends/all+(pewsocialtrends.org+|+All).

41. Robert J. Samuelson, "The Great Recession's Stranglehold," *Washington Post,* July 12, 2010.

42. AARP, *Baby Boomers Envision Their Retirement* (Washington, DC: AARP, February 1999), and *Baby Boomers Envision Retirement II* (Washington, DC: AARP, May 2004); Jack VanDerhei, Sarah Holden, Craig Copeland, and Luis Alonso, "401(k) Plan Asset Allocation, Account Balances, and Loan Activity in 2006," *Employee Benefit Research Institute Issue Brief,* no. 308 (August 2007).

43. Alicia H. Munnell, Anthony Webb, and Luke Delorme, *A New National Retirement Risk Index,* Issue in Brief, no. 48 (Boston: Boston College Center for Retirement Research, June 2006); Diana Farrell and Ezra Greenberg, "Twilight of the Boomers," June 23, 2008, www.economy.com/dismal/article_free.asp?cid=106690&tid=5AB5D93B-6C42-4355-8264-60410C40EF8E. See also Alicia Munnell, Mauricio Soto, Anthony Webb, Francesca Golub-Sass, and Dan Muldoon, *Health Care Costs Drive Up the National Retirement Risk Index,* Issue in Brief, no. 8–3 (Boston: Boston College Retirement Research, 2008); Diana Farrell, Eric Beinhocker, Ezra Greenberg, Suruchi Shukla, Jonathan Ablett, and Geoffrey Green, *Talkin' 'Bout My Generation: The Economic Impact of Aging US Baby Boomers* (San Francisco: McKinsey Global Institute, June 2008).

44. Pew Research Center, "Recession Turns a Graying Office Grayer: America's Changing Workforce," report, September 3, 2009, http://pewsocialtrends.org/pubs/742/americas-changing-work-force#prc-jump.

45. John M. Gibbons, "I Can't Get No . . . Job Satisfaction, That Is: America's Unhappy Workers," Report #1459–09RR, Conference Board, New York,

January 2010, www.conference-board.org/publications/publicationdetail.cfm?
publicationid=1727.

46. Helman et al., "2010 Retirement Confidence Survey."

47. Ibid.

48. Shalanda Gordon, Carol Keegan, and Linda Fisher, "Boomers Turning 60," report, Knowledge Management Group, AARP, 2006, http://assets.aarp .org/rgcenter/general/boomers60.pdf.

49. Joanna Rotenberg, "The Retirement Challenge: Expectations vs. Reality," paper on McKinsey & Company's 2006 Consumer Retirement Survey, presented at the Employee Benefit Research Institute/AARP Pension Conference, May 15, 2006.

50. Employee Benefit Research Institute, *Workers' Retirement Date: Planned vs. Actual,* Fast Facts, no. 129, July 15, 2009. See also Ruth Helman, Mathew Greenwald and Associates, Jack VanDerhei, and Craig Copeland, "The Retirement System in Transition: The 2007 Retirement Confidence Survey," *Employee Benefit Research Institute Issue Brief,* no. 304 (April 2007).

51. Quote from David Wessel, "Older Staffers Get Uneasy Embrace," *Wall Street Journal,* May 15, 2008; see also Alicia Munnell and Steven Sass, *Working Longer* (Washington, DC: Brookings Institution, 2008).

52. Steve Vogel, "Age Discrimination Claims Jump, Worrying EEOC, Worker Advocates," *Washington Post,* July 16, 2009.

53. Julian Mincer, "Getting Personal: Boomers Delay Retirement as Savings Dwindle," *Wall Street Journal,* June 23, 2009; see also Diane Stafford, "Recession Forces More Older Workers to Put Off Retiring," *Kansas City Star,* July 10, 2009.

54. Winerip, "Boomers."

55. Winerip, "Time, It Turns Out."

56. Alicia Munnell, "Retirement Dreams Face New Reality," interview by Kay Ryssdal, *Marketplace,* National Public Radio, May 15, 2009. *High Wire* author Peter Gosselin also doubted boomers' abilities to recoup lost years of retirement savings. Working a few more years into one's sixties is simply too little and too late, Gosselin argued. "It is unlikely that many workers can stay on the job long enough to do more than modestly augment their 401(k)s and other savings arrangements; the mismatch is simply too great between what can be set aside in a few years and how much is needed to support decades of retirement. Moreover, a substantial number of workers will encounter medical or other problems that make continued, full-time work impossible. And

in case you hadn't noticed, most employers are not clamoring for older, more experienced employees; they're pushing for younger, cheaper ones." Peter Gosselin, *High Wire: The Precarious Financial Lives of American Families* (New York: Basic Books, 2008), 28.

57. Edward Yardeni, quoted in Tom Petrumo, "The Case for a New National Frugality," *Los Angeles Times,* August 9, 2008, C1.

58. Ernst and Young issued an equally pessimistic assessment in July 2008—just before the major fall stock market meltdowns. "Many of the 77 million baby boomers retiring over the next few years will face unprecedented challenges in maintaining their standard of living in retirement. Middle-income Americans are most at risk as long life spans, the decline of guaranteed sources of retirement income and the fact that nearly half of older Americans lack employer-based retirement plans contribute to increased retirement risks." Ernst and Young LLP, *Retirement Vulnerability of New Retirees: The Likelihood of Outliving Their Assets* (New York: Ernst and Young, July 2008). One year later, a *Businessweek* cover story acknowledged that many families were frustrated and had a sense of futility about ever trying to achieve recommended levels of retirement savings. Peter Coy, "Can You Afford to Retire?" *Businessweek,* July 2, 2009.

59. *The Metlife Report on Early Boomers* (Westport, CT: Metlife Mature Market Institute/Peter Francese, LLC, September 2010).

60. See Barry Bluestone and Mark Melnick, *After the Recovery: Help Needed* (San Francisco: Civic Ventures, 2010).

61. Daniel Pink, *Free Agent Nation* (New York: Warner Books, 2001).

62. Steven Greenhouse, "Starting Over at 55," *New York Times,* March 3, 2010.

63. Ashlea Ebeling, "Boomers Move to Self-Employment," *Forbes,* July 2, 2009. See also Dane Stangler, *The Coming Entrepreneurship Boom* (Kansas City: Kauffman Foundation. June 2009).

64. Two other upbeat journalistic articles spurred by the Kauffman reports on boomers as potential entrepreneurs are Hanah Cho, "Boomers Go Venturing," *Baltimore Sun,* July 29, 2009, and Elizabeth Razzi, "The Worker's Open Road," *Washington Post,* May 31, 2009.

65. Jeff Goldsmith, *The Long Baby Boom: An Optimistic Vision for a Graying Generation* (Baltimore: Johns Hopkins Press, 2008).

66. "In southern California, nearly 23 percent of telecommuters are in their 50s, compared with only 16.7 percent overall and less than 16 percent of non-teleworkers." Ibid., 85.

67. Laura Vanderkam, "The Promise and Peril of the Freelance Economy," *City Journal* 19, no. 1 (2009), www.city-journal.org/2009/19_1_self-employment .html.

68. See Simona Covel, "Sick and Getting Sicker," *Wall Street Journal,* July 13, 2009.

69. Mark Penn, "Boss Nation," *Wall Street Journal,* August 3, 2009.

70. Richard C. Morais, "The IRA Job Machine," *Forbes,* April 8, 2009.

71. Stephane Fitch, "Gilt-Edged Pensions," *Forbes,* February 16, 2009.

72. Dan Walters, "Pension Fund Setbacks Will Hit Taxpayers Hard," *Sacramento Bee,* January 26, 2009. Indeed, new organizations such as California Pension Reform (www.Californiapensionreform.com) unsuccessfully attempted to gather signatures to curtail future public-sector benefits, while posting on its Web site the members of the "$100k Club"—retired public pensioners who were earning more than $100,000. (The trend is catching on with newspapers around the nation.) See Craig Karmin, "Group Shines Light on Hefty Government Pensions," *Wall Street Journal,* June 24, 2009.

73. John Jannarone, "A Pension Deficit Disorder," *Wall Street Journal,* February 12, 2009.

74. Joe Mont, "Pension Deficits Hit Historic High: $506 Billion," TheStreet.com, September 1, 2010, www.thestreet.com/story/10850461/pension-deficits-hit-historic-high-506-billion.html.

75. See Alicia H. Munnell and Mauricio Soto, "Why Are Companies Freezing Their Pensions?" paper presented at the Ninth Annual Joint Conference of the Retirement Research Consortium, Washington, DC, August 9–10, 2009.

76. Pension Benefit Guaranty Corporation, "Maximum Monthly Guarantee Tables," www.pbgc.gov/ (accessed October 15, 2010).

77. Walt Bogdanich, "A Disability Epidemic among a Railroad's Retirees," *New York Times,* September 21, 2008.

78. Dan Walters, "Pension Hike of a Decade Ago Backfires," *Sacramento Bee,* June 22, 2009.

79. Marc Lifsher, "States Grappling with Pension Fund Deficits," *Los Angeles Times,* February 18, 2010.

80. Michael Barbaro, "Mayor Warns on Pension Costs but Gave Pay Deals," *New York Times,* June 22, 2009.

81. See Roger Lowenstein, "The Next Crisis: Public Pension Funds," *New York Times Magazine,* June 27, 2010.

82. *State and Local Government Retiree Benefits: Current Status of Benefit Structures, Protections and Fiscal Outlook for Funding Future Costs,* GAO-07–1156 (Washington, DC: U.S. Government Accountability Office, September 2007); *State and Local Government Retiree Benefits: Current Funded Status of Pension and Health Benefits,* GAO-08–223 (Washington, DC: U.S. Government Accountability Office, January 2008).

83. Pew Center on the States, *The Trillion Dollar Gap: Underfunded State Retirement Systems and the Roads to Reform,* (Washington, DC: Pew Charitable Trusts, February 2010).

84. Alicia H. Munnell, Jean-Pierre Aubry, and Laura Quinby, *The Funding of State and Local Pensions: 2009–2013,* State and Local Pension Plans, no. 10 (Boston: Boston College Center for Retirement Research, April 2010), 7.

85. See Richard C. Kearney, Robert L. Clark, Jerrell D. Coggburn, Dennis M. Daley, and Christina Robinson, *At a Crossroads: The Financing and Future of Health Benefits for State and Local Government Retirees* (Washington, DC: Center for State and Local Government Excellence, July 2009).

86. Ibid. This report echoed the 2007 Government Accounting Office evaluation warning that states face soaring liabilities for such expenses and cannot continue pay-as-you-go funding from general revenues. See Dennis M. Daley and Jerrell D. Coggburn, *Retiree Health Care in the American States* (Washington, DC: Center for State and Local Government Excellence, December 2008); U.S. General Accounting Office, *State and Local Government Retiree Benefits,* GAO-07–1156 (Washington, DC: U.S. General Accounting Office, September 2007).

87. Steve Lopez, "Deals So Sweet They'll Kill Us," *Los Angeles Times,* January 22, 2006.

88. Evan Halper, "Public Sector Reels at Retiree Healthcare Tab," *Wall Street Journal,* June 10, 2007.

89. See Walsh and Schoenfeld, "Padded Pensions"; Zuckerman, "Bankrupting of America." A *Time* magazine cover story, David von Drehle's "The Broken States of America" (July 28, 2010), highlighted the pension funding crisis, and the reporter Mary Williams Walsh again headlined the problem with "In Budget Crisis, States Take Aim at Pension Costs," *New York Times,* June 10, 2010.

90. See "A Gold-Plated Burden: Hard-Pressed American States Face a Crushing Pensions Bill," *Economist,* October 14, 2010; James A. Bacon Jr., "Will Ballooning State Budgets Be the Next Systemic Financial Crisis?" *Exam-*

iner.com, September 30, 2010. See also R. Eden Martin, "Unfunded Public Pensions—the Next Quagmire," *Wall Street Journal*, August 19, 2010.

91. Evan Halper and Marc Lifsher, "Government Pensions in the Crosshairs," *Los Angeles Times*, April 23, 2010. (That article capped many others in the paper, including an editorial conceding that pension reform had been long overdue. See, for example, "California's Pension Powder Keg," *Los Angeles Times*, August 13, 2009.) See also Jim Christie, "California Pensions Next State Financial Crisis," Reuters, July 29, 2009, www.reuters.com/article/reutersEdge/idUSTRE56S6UB20090729.

92. Matthew Greenwald, interview with the author, September 13, 2007.

93. For a brief, preliminary overview of boomer stereotyping, see H. R. Moody, review of *Aging America and the Boomer Wars*, by Frank J. Whittington, *Gerontologist* 48, no. 6 (2008): 839–44.

94. On the identification of the Clintons, especially Bill Clinton, with boomers, see Howard Fineman, "The Last Hurrah," *Newsweek*, January 23, 2006, 52–61.

95. Howard Fineman, "Boomers: Which Way Will Their Politics Go?" *Newsweek*, August 24, 2007.

96. Peter Feld, "Mark Penn's Missed Microtrends," April 7, 2008, www.portfolio.com/news-markets/top-5/2008/04/07/mr-microtrends-undone-by-microtrends.

97. Frank Rich, "One Historic Night, Two Americas," *New York Times*, June 8, 2008.

98. William Kristol, "Not-So-Great Generation," *Weekly Standard*, November 26, 2007.

99. Michael Barone, "Talkin' 'Bout My Generation: Leaving Boomer Conflicts Behind," *National Review Online*, July 23, 2007, http://article.nationalreview.com/?q=YWJiNTExZmNmN2U2ZjZmZGU3YTQ1NDBhZjI3NWYxODA=.

100. Victor Davis Hansen, "A Generational Bust," *National Review Online*, May 29, 2008, http://article.nationalreview.com/print/?q=NmMwMzM2MDI3MWYwZjI1ODdmMjMiMTE0NjJmNDg4ZDc=.

101. Cathleen Decker, "Whitman Tries to Invoke the '60s," *Los Angeles Times*, June 27, 2010, A35.

102. Cathalena E. Burch, "Black: Baby Boomers Screwed Up," *Arizona Daily Star*, December 31, 2009.

103. Robert J. Samuelson, "Entitled Selfishness: Boomer Generation Is in a State of Denial," *Washington Post*, January 10, 2007.

104. Joe Queenan, *Balsamic Dreams: A Short but Self-Important History of the Baby Boomer Generation* (New York: Picador USA, 2002).

105. Christopher Buckley, *Boomsday* (New York: Twelve/Hachette Book Group, 2007).

106. Meghan Daum, "Why Don't You All Just F-Fade Away?" *Los Angeles Times,* May 25, 2008.

107. Penelope Trunk, "Boomer Kaboomer: What Obama Means for the Workplace," February 7, 2008, www.readthehook.com/code/printStory. aspx?StoryURL=/stories/2008/02/07/BRAZEN-0706-ObamadissesBoomers-A.rtf.aspx.

108. Joel Achenbach, "The Rise of the Alpha Geezer," *Washington Post,* September 9, 2007.

109. See Douglas Belkin, "Boomers to This Year's Grads: We Are Really, Really Sorry," *Wall Street Journal,* June 10, 2009; Mitch Daniels, commencement address at Butler University, May 9, 2009, www.in.gov/portal/news_ events/38894.htm; Sen. Michael Bennet, commencement address to Colorado College class of 2009, www.coloradocollege.edu/Commencement/Michael-Bennet.asp.

110. Nicholas D. Kristof, "Geezers Doing Good," *New York Times,* July 20, 2008.

111. Michael Kinsley, "It's the Least We Can Do," *Atlantic Monthly,* October 2010. See also the reflections of British baby boomer Will Hutton, who wonders if his generation was "lucky" and states that children now face a "future of massive debt and uncertainty." Will Hutton, "The Baby Boomers and the Price of Personal Freedom," *Guardian,* August 22, 2010.

112. Stephen Moore, "This Boomer Isn't Going to Apologize," *Wall Street Journal,* June 16, 2009.

113. John Zogby, "The Baby Boomers' Legacy," *Forbes,* July 23, 2009.

114. See Perry Bacon Jr. and Shailagh Murry, "Opponents Paint Obama as an Elitist," *Washington Post,* April 12, 2008.

115. Frank Rich, "She Broke the G.O.P. and Now She Owns It," *New York Times,* July 12, 2009.

116. Maureen Dowd, "Sarah's Ghoulish Carousel," *New York Times,* August 16, 2009.

117. Richard Cohen, "Palin's Red Menace," *Washington Post,* August 18, 2009.

118. Phillip Longman, "After the Boom," *Atlantic Monthly,* January 2008.

119. Ibid.

120. Harris Interactive Survey, "Widely Held Attitudes to Different Generations," press release, August 20, 2008, www.harrisinteractive.com/news/allnewsbydate.asp?NewsID=1328.

121. Paul Taylor and Richard Morin, "Forty Years after Woodstock, a Gentler Generation Gap," Social and Democratic Trends Report, Pew Research Center, August 12, 2009, http://pewsocialtrends.org/assets/pdf/after-woodstock-gentler-generation-gap.pdf.

122. Rich Morin, "Black-White Conflict Isn't Society's Largest: The Public Assesses Social Divisions," Social and Democratic Trends Report, Pew Research Center, September 24, 2009, http://pewsocialtrends.org/pubs/744/social-divisions-black-white-conflict-not-society-largest-.

5. NOT YOUR FATHER'S AARP

The chapter's epigraph is from Dale Van Atta, "This Isn't the Old AARP," *Los Angeles Times,* July 4, 2006.

1. Center for Responsive Politics, "Lobbying Top Spenders," 2003–8, www.opensecrets.org/lobby/top.php?showYear+a&indexType+s.

2. Simpson continued his war against AARP after retiring from the Senate in 2000. "AARP could be such a force for good . . . but they're not. They're selfish, greedy. They don't care about their grandchildren a whit. . . . Now I have the freedom to just beat the brains out of the AARP and I do that all over America." Alan Simpson, "Let 'er Rip! Reflections of a Rocky Mountain Senator," transcript and Webcast, Conversations with History, Institute of International Studies, University of California, Berkeley, 1997, http://globetrotter.berkeley.edu/conversations/Simpson/.

3. See Charles R. Morris, *The AARP: America's Most Powerful Lobby and the Clash of Generations* (New York: Times Books, 1996), and Dale Van Atta, *Trust Betrayed: Inside the AARP* (Washington, DC: Regnery, 1998).

4. Rich Tau, telephone interview with the author, February 21, 2007.

5. AARP Public Policy Institute, "2009 Annual Report: Together Creating Opportunities," http://assets.aarp.org/www.aarp.org/cs/misc/aarp_annual_report_2009.pdf, 10.

6. See Charles R. Morris, *The AARP* (New York: Times Books, 1996), 105–13.

7. Rich Tau, telephone interview with the author, February 21, 2007.

8. "Jabba the AARP," *Wall Street Journal,* May 17, 1999, A26.

9. "AARP: Making Money, Losing Trust," Bloomberg News Service, January 15, 2009.

10. Ibid.

11. My analysis of the changes wrought by Novelli at AARP is based upon dozens of interviews and reinterviews with staff and researchers at various levels of the organization, including two interviews with Novelli (on December 12, 2000, and December 5, 2007). Although there are no current books or academic journal articles on AARP's Novelli-led transformation, there is one major unpublished professional paper and several first-rate journalistic sources. Dartmouth's Tuck Business School Professor Paul A. Argenti authored an in-house account entitled "AARP: At the Crossroads of Change," unpublished manuscript, AARP and Tuck Business School, 2005. Two key articles in *National Journal* are Bara Vaida, "AARP's Big Bet," *National Journal,* March 13, 2004, and Julie Kosterlitz, "The World According to AARP," *National Journal,* March 10, 2007, 28–35. See also Jane Eisinger Rooney, "Brand New Day," *Association Management 55,* no. 2 (2003): 46–48, 50–51.

12. See Bill Novelli, *50+: Igniting a Revolution to Reinvent America* (New York: St. Martin's Press, 2006).

13. See "Our Leadership," under "About AARP," www.aarp.org/about-aarp/.

14. Bill Novelli, "Moving AARP Ahead: From Good to Great," July 25, 2005, www.aarp.org.

15. Bill Novelli, telephone interview with the author, July 1, 2010.

16. Vaida, "AARP's Big Bet."

17. Bill Novelli, interview with the author, December 5, 2007, Washington, DC.

18. See AARP, "Mission," under "About AARP," 2001, www.aarp.org/about-aarp; AARP, *Reimagining America: How American Can Grow Older and Prosper* (Washington, DC: AARP Publications, 2005).

19. See Argenti, "AARP."

20. See "Consolidated Financial Statements" section of AARP, *2009 Annual Report* (Washington, DC: AARP, 2010). Conservative critics grumble that in 2008 AARP received about ninety million dollars in government funds through its affiliated, charitable AARP Foundation to administer free tax consulting and job training for senior citizens. The 2008 donor list mentions "institutional support" from the Internal Revenue Service, the Department of Health and Human Services, the Department of Housing and Urban Development, and the Department of Labor. See Chelsea Schilling, "Dark Secrets of AARP Finally Exposed to Light," *World Net Daily,* November 10, 2009, www.wnd.com/?pageId=115617.

21. Andrew Adam Newman, "A Magazine Now Tailored to the Not Necessarily Retired," *New York Times*, August 23, 2010; also Richard Siklos, "At Some Publishers, Nonbusiness Is Going Strong," *New York Times*, August 20, 2006; Marc Fisher, "AARP Tunes In to Radio's Discarded Audience," *Washington Post*, July 8, 2007; Andrew Billups, "AARP Magazine Targets 'New 50,'{hrs}" *Washington Times*, October 29, 2007; Elaine S. Povich, "AARP the Magazine Online Feature Wins 2009 National Magazine Award," *AARP Bulletin Today*, May 1, 2009.

22. See AARP, "AARP Global Network Expands International Reach," press release, February 28, 2008, http://share-ws2-md.aarp.org/aarp/presscenter/pressrelease/articles/aarp_global_network_expands_international_reach.html.

23. AARP, "Audience Demographics," in "Life at 50+: Sponsor and Exhibitor Prospectus," Washington, DC, 2008, 5. Also "Who We Are: Profile of AARP's 40 Million Members," *AARP Bulletin*, June 2009.

24. "AARP Member Demographics Study," 2008, internal document.

25. Barbara T. Dreyfuss, "The Seduction," *American Prospect*, June 6, 2007.

26. AARP's backing of the Medicare Modernization Act attracted a good deal of notice and commentary. See Laurie McGinley, "AARP Chief under Fire on the Medicare Bill," *Wall Street Journal*, November 20, 2003; Robert Pear and David E. Rosenbaum, "AARP Backs Republican Plan for Medicare Drug Benefits," *New York Times*, November 17, 2003; David S. Broder and Amy Goldstein, "AARP Decision Followed a Long GOP Courtship," *Washington Post*, November 20, 2003; David S. Broder, "AARP's Tough Selling Job," *Washington Post*, March 18, 2004; Dale Van Atta, "This Isn't the Old AARP," *Los Angeles Times*, November 24, 2003; "Fading Senior Support?" *Newsweek*, October 25, 2004. For an interesting observation on the role of aging boomers in AARP's Medicare decision, see Sheryl Gay Stolberg and Milt Freudenheim, "AARP Support for Medicare Bill Came as Group Grew 'Younger,'" *New York Times*, November 26, 2003. For one of Novelli's many published explanations on the Medicare decision, see William D. Novelli, "AARP Stays Sharp," *Wall Street Journal*, December 4, 2003.

27. According to one AARP source, the American business establishment was fearful of tampering with Social Security and only reluctantly supported the Bush administration private accounts initiative. Still, one major business magazine raised the questions of whether AARP's commercial and political interests were in potential conflict—and whether many of their sponsored

products represented the best value for seniors. See "By Raising Its Voice, AARP Raises Questions," *Businessweek,* March 14, 2005.

28. "AARP Criticized over Health Plans," editorial, *Des Moines Register,* April 24, 2009; see also Robert Pear, "AARP Orders Investigation Concerning Its Marketing," *New York Times,* November 19, 2008.

29. See Bob Trebilcock's series "AARP Funds: Is AARP Looking Out for You?" (Mutual Funds, July 9, 2009; Life Insurance and Annuities, August 5, 2009; Auto and Homeowners Insurance, August 26, 2009; Health and Long Term Care Insurance, October 9, 2008), all at CBS Moneywatch.com, http://moneywatch.bnet.com/retirement-planning/feature/is-aarp-looking-out-for-you/351187/?tag=video-351895;related-link-2.

30. Charles Morris, *The AARP* (New York: Times Books, 1996), 58.

31. These quotes are from the 2006 Strategic Plan—representative of an evolving document about midway through Novelli's transformative reign.

32. AARP's coveted public trust was damaged recently via a lawsuit and subsequent congressional hearings claiming that some AARP-endorsed high-deductible health insurance policies (through United Health Care) did not provide adequate catastrophic coverage; see Pear, "AARP Orders Investigation." In addition, a widely circulated article by Bloomberg News Service called attention to AARP's rake-off from the comparatively high prices of insurance products endorsed and sold by the organization. See Gary Bohn and Darrell Preston, "AARP Gets a Cut of Policies It Endorses: Insurance Prices Are Called Inflated Because of Royalties," *Detroit Free Press,* December 7, 2008.

33. Simpson, "Let 'er Rip!"

34. On the AARP's increasingly aggressive "business" persona, see Claudia H. Deutsch, "AARP Wants You (to Buy Its Line of Products)," *New York Times,* October 28, 2005.

35. John Rother had been active in getting AARP to prepare for the boomers before Bill Novelli arrived. On these early efforts, see Susan Levine, "AARP Hopes Boom Times Are Ahead," *Washington Post,* June 2, 1998; also David J. Lipke, "Fountain of Youth: AARP Woos Reluctant Boomers with High-Priced Makeover," *American Demographics* 22 (September 2000): 37–40.

36. Robert Samuelson, "AARP's America Is a Mirage," *Washington Post,* July 4, 2006.

37. Proceeds from the books sales went to the AARP Foundation.

38. AARP, *Reimagining America,* 1.

39. The preface of *Reimagining America* states: "AARP believes that as a nation we can balance longer lives with the pressures of the aging of the boomers and increased longevity put on our social systems. While this is often described as a confounding problem of demographics, it is actually driven by the fragmented and disorganized delivery of health care which costs too much and delivers to little."

40. AARP, *Reimagining America*, 19.

41. *Reimagining America's* boldface preface declares: "We also believe that solutions must come from collaboration among government, private organizations, and individuals."

42. Ibid., 3.

43. Ibid., 19.

44. Christopher Buckley wrote about this encounter with Shepherd in "I Dream of Cybill Shepherd . . . ," *Wall Street Journal*, November 2, 2004.

45. The October 2005 conference scheduled for New Orleans was canceled because of Hurricane Katrina.

46. Jody Holtzman, interview with the author, December 5, 2007, Washington, DC.

47. Joanne Handy, Jennie Chin Hansen, and John Rother, "Reimagining America's Healthcare: AARP Targets Healthcare Reform" and "How to Talk to the American Public about Health Reform: Results of AARP Message Research," joint presentations at the annual meetings of the American Society on Aging/National Conference on Aging, Chicago, March 7, 2007.

48. Pew Research Center, "No Post-Trip Bounce for Obama: Inflation Staggers Public, Economy Still Seen as Fixable," report, July 31, 2008, http://people-press.org/reports/pdf/438.pdf 6.

49. U. S. Census Bureau, "An Older and More Diverse Nation by Midcentury," press release, August 14, 2008, www.census.gov/newsroom/releases/archives/population/cb08–123.html; see also Conor Dougherty, "Whites to Lose Majority Status in the U.S. by 2042," *Wall Street Journal*, August 14, 2008, A3.

50. "AARP Ethel Percy Andrus Legacy Awards," 2008, www.aarp.org/aarp/articles/the_aarp_ethel_percy.html.

6. AARP TURNS FIFTY

1. Bill Novelli, interview with the author, Washington, DC, December 5, 2007.

2. AARP was also active in lobbying for the Serve America Act, designed to boost philanthropic and nonprofit organizations' efforts to promote civic participation and volunteering.

3. Michael Winerip, telephone interview with the author, July 18, 2008.

4. Paul Briand, telephone interview with the author, August 3, 3009.

5. Kevin Bogardus, "AARP and Business Groups Lobby Hard for Bailout Package," *The Hill,* October 1, 2008, http://thehill.com/business-a-lobbying/3756-aarp-and-business-groups-lobby-hard-for-bailout-package.

6. "AARP Congressional Awards Program," February 19, 2009, www.aarp.org/makeadifference/advocacy/GovernmentWatch/articles/congressional_awards.html.

7. "2008 AARP Voters Guide," *AARP Magazine,* September/October 2008, 93–98.

8. A 2006 AARP National Member Survey about election issues found that 90 percent supported allowing Medicare to use its bargaining power to lower prices for prescription drugs; 81 percent opposed using Social Security taxes to fund private accounts; 72 percent supported a shared approach whereby the federal government, employers, and individuals together would pay for providing health care coverage for everyone; 69 percent supported a shared approach that would involve both government and individuals paying for long-term care; and 66 percent opposed changing the traditional Medicare program by imposing an annual limit on federal Medicare spending. "AARP National Member Survey about 2006 Election Issues," June 26, 2006, http://assets.aarp.org/rgcenter/general/election_2006.pdf.

9. AARP did resist George W. Bush's efforts to establish private Social Security accounts. And Bill Novelli and John Rother have urgently warned about problems in risk-shift retirement—as they did in the prescient PBS *Frontline* documentary "Can You Afford to Retire?" May 16, 2006.

10. See A. Barry Rand, "Where We Stand: Health Reform Now," *AARP Bulletin,* July–August 2009, 26.

11. Alicia Mundy and Laura Meckler, "Drug Makers Score Early Wins as Plan Takes Shape," *Wall Street Journal,* July 17, 2009.

12. Ibid.

13. Reader comment on "Bill Novelli on the Financial Summit," ShAARP Session, February 2009, http://blog.aarp.org/shaarpsession/2009/02/aarp_ceo_bill_novelli_reports.html.

14. Rachel Martin and Jake Tapper, "President Obama's 'Senior' Moment," Political Punch, August 2009, http://blogs.abcnews.com/political

punch/2009/08/president-obamas-senior-moment.html. (Several responses to the ABC News Web site reports indicated cancellation of AARP memberships.)

15. "Health Care Reform and You," *New York Times,* July 26, 2009.

16. John Rother, interview, *The Rachel Maddow Show,* MSNBC, August 11, 2009.

17. Reader comment on "Town Hall Meeting on Health Care Reform for Older Americans," *AARP Bulletin,* July 17, 2009, http://bulletin.aarp.org/yourhealth/policy/articles/town_hall_meeting_on_health_care_reform_for_older_americans.html.

18. Reader comment on "Bipartisan Group Eyes Medicare Savings," *AARP Bulletin,* July 28, 2009, http://bulletin.aarp.org/yourhealth/medicare/articles/ap_sources_bipartisan_group _eyes_medicare_savings.comments.o.html.

19. Mark Tapscot, "Obamacare Could Kill AARP," *Washington Examiner,* July 30, 2009, www.washingtonexaminer.com/opinion/columns/Obamacare-could-kill-AARP-8036046–51988312.html; Drew Nannis, "AARP: Setting the Record Straight," *Washington Examiner,* August 5, 2009, www.washingtonexaminer.com/opinion/columns/OpEd-Contributor/AARP-Setting-the-record-straight-52105997.html.

20. One of the most devastating early critiques of the proposals was written by a former Clinton health care reform opponent, Betsy McCaughey, "GovernmentCare's Assault on Seniors," *Wall Street Journal,* July 23, 2006. This article was the primary target of John Rother's rebuttals in "AARP Responds to Health Reform Scare Tactics," AARP press release, July 24, 2009.

21. Frank Newport, "Americans on Healthcare Reform: Top 10 Takeaways," Gallup Poll, July 31, 2009, www.gallup.com/poll/121997/americans-healthcare-reform-top-takeaways.aspx.

22. Ann Flaherty, "Emails from Public Overload House Web Site," Associated Press, August 13, 2009, http://apnews.myway.com/article/20090813/D9A25N781.html.

23. Ceci Connolly, "Seniors Remain Wary of Health-Care Reform," *Washington Post,* August 9, 2009.

24. Paul Steinhauser, "Poll Indicates Generational Split over Health Care," CNN, August 5, 2009, www.cnn.com/2009/POLITICS/08/05/health.care.poll/index.html; also CNN Opinion Research Poll, August 4, 2008, http://i.cdn.turner.com/cnn/2009/images/08/04/rel11b.pdf. A Gallup poll also found that those over age sixty-five were far less likely than other age groups to perceive that the new health care legislation would improve their medical care (Newport, "Americans on Healthcare Reform").

25. Pew Research Center, "Obama's Ratings Slide across the Board," Section 4, "Health Care Overhaul," July 30, 2009, http://people-press.org/report/532/obamas-ratings-slide. Americans over sixty-five were among those "very closely" following the issue (56 percent), as were college graduates (57 percent), those earning more than $75,000 (55 percent), and Republicans (56 percent). Conversely, the least interested were age eighteen to thirty-nine (37 percent), high school graduate or less (35 percent), and below $30,000 (32 percent). Half of boomers (age forty to sixty-four) were "very interested," as were 46 percent of political independents and 42 percent of Democrats. Pew Research Center, "Many Fault Media Coverage of Health Care Debate," report, August 6, 2009, http://people-press.org/report/533/many-fault-media-coverage-of-health-care. See also Charles M. Blow, "Health Care Hullaballoo," *New York Times,* August 8, 2009.

26. "NBC News Health Care Survey," August 2009, http://msnbcmedia.msn.com/i/MSNBC/Sections/NEWS/NBC-WSJ_Poll.pdf.

27. Miriam Jordan, "Illegal Immigration Enters the Health-Care Debate," *Wall Street Journal,* August 15, 2009.

28. "Illegal Immigrants Debate Could Potentially Block Reform," editorial, *Los Angeles Times,* August 17, 2009.

29. Ronald Brownstein, "The New Color Line," *National Journal,* October 10, 2009.

30. Thomas Edsall, "Ghost Story: Realignment Was Just an Illusion," *New Republic,* January 20, 2010.

31. Ronald Brownstein, "Dems Caught in Populist Crossfire," *National Journal,* March 27, 2010.

32. Jonathan Weisman, "Middle Class Starts to Drift from Obama," *Wall Street Journal,* March 26, 2010.

33. Peter Brown, "Like Affirmative Action, Arizona Law Splits Elites and the Public," *Wall Street Journal,* May 20, 2010. And, again, see Damien Cave, "A Generation Gap over Immigration," *New York Times,* May 17, 2010.

34. Dave Cook, "Healthcare Reform Has Turned into a Roller Derby, AARP Says," *Christian Science Monitor,* October 14, http://features.csmonitor.com/politics/2009/10/14heatlhcare-reform-has-turned-into-a-roller-derby-AARP-says.

35. Dan Eggen, "AARP: Reform Advocate and Insurance Salesman," *Washington Post,* October 27, 2009.

36. Gardiner Harris, "A Heated Debate Is Dividing Generations in AARP," *New York Times,* October 4, 2009.

37. National Public Radio/Kaiser Family Foundation/Harvard School of Public Health, "Survey on the Role of Health Care Interest Groups," September 2009, www.npr.org/assets/news/health/2009/09/poll/topline.pdf. See also Peter Overby, "Conflict of Interest for ARP in Health Bill Debate?" National Public Radio, *Morning Edition,* November 4, 2009, www.npr.org/templates/story/story.php?storyId=120069183.

38. "53% Have Favorable Opinion of AARP, but Health Care Issue Hurting Reputation," Rasmussen Reports, November 29, 2009, www.rasmussenreports.com/public_content/politics/current_events/healthcare/november_2009/53_have_favorable_opinion_of_aarp_but_health_care_issue_hurting_reputation.

39. "I Joined the New AARP!" January 17, 2010, Here's My View on It!, http://moneyback1234.blogspot.com2010/011-joined-new-aarp.html.

40. Ronald Brownstein, "The Other Health Care Story," *National Journal,* September 5, 2009.

41. Timothy J. Burger, "Obama Campaign Ad Firms Signed On to Push Health-Care Overhaul," August 15, 2009, www.bloomberg.com/apps/news?pid=newsarchive&sid=aV3dLt6wmZH4.

42. Their new documentary *I.O.U.S.A.: The Movie* (dir. Patrick Creadon, prod. Christine O'Malley, 2008) gained critical attention during its run in theaters and has been aired subsequently as a two-hour weekend special on CNN, where Walker has become a frequent analyst.

43. On the "Blue Dog Democrats," see Christopher Hayes, "Blue Dogs Bark," *Nation,* February 11, 2009. Also within this same fiscally conservative orbit is a recently revived Americans for Generational Equity, founded and still guided extensively by Paul Hewitt, former George W. Bush appointee as Social Security Administration undersecretary and, before that, director of the Center for Strategic and International Studies' Global Aging Program.

44. See James Ruttenberg, "Liberal Groups Are Flexing New Muscle in Lobby Wars," *New York Times,* March 1, 2009.

45. Peter Wallsten, "Retooling Obama's Campaign Machine for the Long Haul," *Los Angeles Times,* January 14, 2009. See also Eric Etheridge, "Obama 2.0: Who's Leading Who?" *New York Times,* January 16, 2009; Steve Benan, "The Political Animal," *Washington Monthly,* January 14, 2009; "Obama Musters Campaign Army for Economic Fight," Breitbart.com, March 9, 2009, www.breitbart.com/article.php?id=CNG.1da91b565bedacc6461ea17550408182.661&show_article=1; Peter Slevin and Michael Laris, "Obama's Army on Road Again," *Washington Post,* March 22, 2009, A01; Harold Meyerson, "An Army

Untapped," *Washington Post,* July 8, 2009; Peter Wallstein, "Obama's Ground Level of Supporters Put to the Test," *Los Angeles Times,* August 10, 2009; Eli Saslow, "Grass-Roots Battle Tests the Obama Movement," *Washington Post,* August 23, 2009.

46. Maureen Dowd, "Toilet Paper Barricades," *New York Times,* August 12, 2009.

47. John Rother, interview with the author, Washington, DC, June 2, 2010.

48. Nearly a week after my conversation with Rother about "reinvention," a *Wall Street Journal* article noted the trend toward "reinvention" in late middle age—but with some sobering warnings. See Neil Parmar, "Middle Age Crazy? It'll Cost You To Do Your Own Thing," *Wall Street Journal,* June 13, 2010.

49. Alicia Williams, John Fries, Jean Koppen, and Robert Prisuta, "Connecting and Giving: A Report on How Mid-life and Older Americans Spend Their Time, Make Connections and Build Communities," AARP report, January 2010, www.aarp.org/giving-back/volunteering/info-01–2010/connecting_giving.html.

50. Scott Harrington, a professor of health care management at the University of Pennsylvania's Wharton School, concluded that AARP's willingness to support Medicare cuts in order to expand insurance to younger Americans was likely the result of "the organization's reform agenda [that] reflects the progressive/liberal views of a leadership willing to risk alienating many members and prospective members in pursuing its vision." "The AARP Paradox," *The American* (Journal of the American Enterprise Institute), October 2009, www.american/com/archive/2009/October/the-aarp-paradox/article.html.

7. YOU CAN'T ALWAYS GET WHAT YOU WANT

Chapter epigraphs are from David Brooks, "A Date with Scarcity," *New York Times,* November 4, 2008, and Brett Arends, "A Nation of Helen Thomases," *Wall Street Journal,* June 11, 2010.

1 Carleen MacKay, interview with the author, June 30, 2009.

2. Focalyst, *Yesterday, Today, and Tomorrow: Understanding Boomer Segments,* Focalyst Insight Report, February 2009, www.focalyst.com/Sites/Focalyst/Media/Pdfs/en/CurrentResearchReports/6808CC5C.pdf.

3. Peggy Noonan, "Remembering the Dawn of the Age of Abundance," *Wall Street Journal,* February 20, 2009.

4. Quoted in Deborah Gage, "Context for Startups That Help Aging Boomers," *San Francisco Chronicle,* June 18, 2009. The survey Holzman directed,

S. Kathi Brown's *A Year-End Look at the Economic Slowdown's Impact on Middle-Aged and Older Americans* (Washington, DC: AARP Knowledge Management. January 2009), found that 68 percent had reduced entertainment spending and 64 percent had cut back on eating out; more seriously, 52 percent had difficulty paying for essential items such as food, gas, and medicine.

5. Boomers' status as a recognizable sociological entity with a latent political identity (divided by subgroups) is strikingly similar to C. Wright Mills's description sixty ago of a large, emerging "new middle class" of salaried office workers, salespeople, and professionals. Like the boomers, this growing occupational class was important because of its sheer size and because its development was unanticipated; white-collar workers were neither "proletariat" nor "bourgeoisie." Mills found few signs of emerging white-collar class consciousness or political action by this large and potentially powerful entity. He might have been writing about today's aging baby boomers when he stated, "They are diversified in social form, contradictory in material interest, dissimilar in ideological illusion; there is no homogeneity of base among them for a common political movement." C. Wright Mills, *White Collar* (New York: Oxford University Press, 1951), 351–52.

6. Carleen MacKay, interview with the author, June 30, 2009.

7. *Early Boomers: How America's Leading Edge Baby Boomers Will Transform Aging, Work and Retirement* (Westport, CT: Metlife Mature Market Institute/ Peter Francese, LLC, September 2010).

8. On how "one legacy of the Great Recession is that insecurity and uncertainty have gone upscale," see Robert Samuelson, "The Great Recession's Stranglehold," *Washington Post,* July 12, 2010.

9. MacKay, interview with author, June 30, 2009.

10. After the 2008 elections, gentry boomers on the Obama White House staff launched a media campaign to set Republican gentry against middle- and working-class so-called "Walmart Republicans" by attempting to label polarizing conservative radio talk show host Rush Limbaugh as the "Voice of the Republican Party." And the 2009 HBO documentary *Right Americans—Feeling Wronged* is a typical exercise in stereotyping—though not necessarily confined to boomers.

11. Kate Zernike and Megan Thee-Brenan, "Poll Finds Tea Party Backers Wealthy and More Educated," *New York Times,* April 14, 2010. A subsequent Bloomberg national poll of Tea Party supporters found that 53 percent would consider raising the eligibility age for Medicare and 58 percent would consider similar action on Social Security—compared to 47 percent and 49

percent, respectively, of the general public. These are more modest reforms; the question of cutting benefits was not asked. See Lisa Lerer, "Poll: Tea Party Economic Gloom Fuels Republican Momentum," October 13, 2010, www .bloomberg.com/news/2010–10–14/tea-party-s-economic-gloom-fuels-repub-lican-election-momentum-poll-says.html. Also see a *New York Times* profile of a boomer couple who attended a Georgia town hall meeting by Kevin Sack, "Calm, but Moved to Be Heard on Health Care," *New York Times*, August 25, 2009.

12. Paul Briand, interview with the author, August 4, 2009.

13. Robert B. Reich, *Supercapitalism* (New York: Alfred A. Knopf, 2007).

14. Robert Putnam, "*E Pluribus Unum:* Diversity and Community in the Twenty-First Century: The 2006 Joan Skytte Prize Lecture," *Scandinavian Political Studies* 30, no. 2 (2007): 137–74.

15. One partial exception to this silence was a September 2008 panel discussion hosted by AARP International, entitled "Immigration: Challenges, Trends, and the Impact on the U.S. Labor Force," www.aarpinternational.org/resourcelibrary/resourcelibrary_show.htm?doc_id=805430. Along with a one-time partnership with the National Council of LaRaza to educate elderly Hispanics and their families on the Medicare prescription drug program, the tone of the panel discussion and some other statements about a "universal approach to social problems" suggested to *World Net Daily* reporter Chelsea Schilling a latent AARP proimmigration entitlement tilt. See Chelsea Schilling, "Dark Secrets of AARP Finally Exposed to Light," *World Net Daily*, May 14, 2010.

16. See Steven A. Camarota, Robert Rector, Mark Krikorian, and James R. Edwards Jr., "The Elephant in the Room: Panel on Immigration's Impact on Health Care Reform," Washington, DC, Center for Immigration Studies, August 2009, www.cis.org/Transcript/HealthCare-Immigration-Panel.

17. See Alan Berube et al., *State of Metropolitan America* (Washington, DC: Brookings Institution, 2010).

18. For example, see John M. Bridgeland, Robert D. Putnam, and Harris L. Wofford, *More to Give: Tapping the Talents of the Baby Boomer, Silent and Greatest Generations,* report by Civic Enterprises in association with Peter D. Hart Research Associates (Washington, DC: AARP, September 2008). For assessments of boomers and civic engagement before the 2008 economic turmoil, see Laura B. Wilson and Sharon Simson, eds., *Civic Engagement and the Baby Boom Generation* (Binghamton, NY: Haworth Press, 2006).

19. J. Walker Smith and Ann Clurman, *Generation Ageless* (New York: HarperCollins, 2007), 213.

20. Ibid., 165.

21. Anonymous source, interview with the author, March 5, 2009.

22. Alicia Williams, John Fries, Jean Koppen, and Robert Prisuta, "Connecting and Giving: A Report on How Mid-life and Older Americans Spend Their Time, Make Connections and Build Communities," AARP report, January 2010, www.aarp.org/giving-back/volunteering/info-01–2010/connecting_giving.html.

23. Jeff Opdyke, "Who Will Pay for College?" *Wall Street Journal,* August 16, 2008.

24. See Robert Nisbet, *The Sociological Tradition* (New York: Basic Books, 1966).

25. Brian Williams, on *The Rachel Maddow Show,* MSNBC, July 17, 2009.

26. Andrew Kohut, "Would Americans Welcome Medicare if It Were Being Proposed in 2009?" Pew Research Center, August 19, 2009, http://pewresearch.org/pubs/1317/would-americans-welcome-medicare-if-proposed-in-2009.

27. William A. Galston and Elaine C. Kamarck, "Change You Can Believe In Needs a Government You Can Trust," Third Way Report, Washington, DC, November 2008, http://content.thirdway.org/publications/133/Third_Way_Report_-_Trust_in_Government.pdf.

28. Elaine C. Kamarck, "The Evolving American State: The Trust Challenge," *Forum* 7, no. 4 (2009), art. 9.

29. Jason Zweig, "Will We Ever Trust Wall Street Again?" *Wall Street Journal,* February 7, 2010.

30. Paul Volcker, on *The Charlie Rose Show,* September 30, 2009, www.charlierose.com/view/interview/10635#frame_top.

31. Frank Luntz, "What Americans Really Want," *Los Angeles Times,* September 27, 2009.

32. Pew Research Center, "The People and Their Government: Distrust, Discontent, Anger and Partisan Rancor," report, April 18, 2010, http://people-press.org/reports/pdf/606.pdf. The Pew Center report was published on the heels of almost the exact same findings in a February 2010 New York Times/CBS News poll that found that only 19 percent of respondents felt they could trust the government to do the right thing "always" (3 percent) or "most of the time" (16 percent); conversely 81 percent responded "never" (7 percent) or "some of the time" (74 percent)—tied with 1995 as the lowest trust level since the poll began in 1976. New York Times/CBS News Poll, February 5–10, 2010, http://graphics8.nytimes.com/packages/images/nytint/docs/new-york-times-cbs-news-poll/original.pdf.

33. Don Peck, "How a New Jobless Era Will Transform America," *Atlantic Monthly*, March 2010.

34. AARP, *A Changing Political Landscape as One Generation Replaces Another* (Washington, DC: AARP Knowledge Management, 2004), 14.

35. Ibid., 13.

36. Thomas J. Friedman, "The Fat Lady Has Sung," *New York Times*, February 21, 2010; the call for regeneration was issued again in Thomas J. Friedman's "Root Canal Politics," *New York Times*, May 8, 2010.

37. David Brooks, "The Geezers' Crusade," *New York Times*, February 2, 2010.

38. Casey B. Mulligan, "Are We Overpaying Grandpa?" *New York Times*, February 24, 2010.

39. See Lerer, "Poll."

40. "Mixed Views of GOP Proposals on Entitlements," press release, Pew Research Center, September 13, 2010, http://pewresearch.org/pubs/1726/poll-social-security-medicare-republican-plans-bush-tax-cuts-gop-leader.

41. See Tara Siegel Bernard, "Social Security Jitters? Better Prepare Now," *New York Times*, July 31, 2010; "Our View on Social Security: To Shore It Up, Raise the Retirement Age," *USA Today*, September 22, 2010; and "Dealing with Deficits," *Los Angeles Times*, October 16, 2010; "Our View on Social Security: Do a Favor for the Grandkids and Don't Give Seniors a Raise," *USA Today*, October 21, 2010; Nancy LeaMond, "Opposing View on Social Security: Seniors Need Relief to Keep Up," *USA Today*, October 20, 2010; Ronald Brownstein, "Misplaced Zinger," *National Journal*, October 21, 2010.

42. Fareed Zakaria, "How to Restore the American Dream," *Time*, November 1, 2010.

43. For example, see Bill Galston and Maya MacGuineas, "The Future Is Now: A Balanced Plan to Stabilize the Public Debt and Promote Economic Growth," September 30, 2010, http://crfb.org/document/future-now-plan-stabilize-public-debt-and-promote-economic-growth.

44. See a remarkable "AARP Solutions Forum" panel discussion that includes AARP's John Rother, the retirement economist Alicia Munnell (cited frequently in this book), Alice Rivlin (a Brookings Institution senior fellow), and other experts: "Social Security and the Future of Retirement," September 22, 2010, http://assets.aarp.org/rgcenter/ppi/econ-sec/transcript-092210.pdf.

45. Again see Michael Kinsley, "It's the Least We Can Do," *Atlantic Monthly*, October 2010, and the online forum on Kinsley's article "exploring the legacy of the Baby Boomers and what they owe the country."

INDEX

AARP: appeal to baby boomers, 4, 6, 144–46, 147–49, 150, 152, 251 n.35; center-left political persona, 171–74, 184, 253 n.8; civic engagement campaigns, 198; coalition-building, 184–86, 206, 256 n.43; commercial trust brand, 136, 142, 143, 173, 176, 182–83, 188, 190; conservative criticisms of, 71–72, 131, 132–33, 144, 175, 248 n.2, 249 n.20; diversity mission, 138–39, 162–65, 168–69, 172; liberal criticisms of, 135, 140–42, 173–74, 175; "Life @ 50+" conferences, 1–2, 6–7, 8–9, 135, 139, 141, 152–58, 166–69; mission of, 129–30; name change, 3, 130–31; Novelli background, 133–34; origins of, 130–31; power of, 132–33; reorganization, 131–32; role in senior power potential, 3, 72, 196–97; Rother background, 146–47. *See also* AARP consumer services; AARP policies on health care; AARP policies on Social Security/Medicare; AARP social policies; AARP warrior brand; "Life @ 50+" conferences

"AARP: Making Money, Losing Trust" (Bloomberg News), 142
AARP: The Magazine, 145–46
AARP Bulletin, 138
AARP consumer services: and AARP mission, 129–30; criticisms of, 142, 250–51 nn.27,32; and economic anxieties, 158–59; and rebranding, 4, 137; and reorganization, 131; and trust image, 136; and warrior brand, 136–37, 143, 144
AARP Financial Services, 131, 137
AARP Foundation, 131, 249 n.20
AARP Grassroots America, 131–32, 171, 179
AARP Magazine, 137–38, 172
AARP policies on health care: and AARP blueprint publications, 151; and age/race divide, 175; conservative criticisms of, 4, 175; and diversity mission, 164; "Divided We Fail" campaign, 15, 130, 139, 158–63, 166, 169–70, 179, 189; liberal criticisms of, 4, 173–74, 175; Medicare Modernization Act, 71, 141, 250 n.26; and presidential election (2008), 162–63, 171; and rebranding,

263

Text:	10.75/15 Janson
Display:	Janson MT Pro
Compositor:	Toppan Best-set Premedia Limited
Indexer:	Do Mi Stauber
Printer and binder:	Maple-Vail Book Manufacturing Group